Radiotherapy in Practice

Radiotherapy in Practice
Physics for clinical oncology

SECOND EDITION

Edited by

Amen Sibtain
Consultant Clinical Oncologist, Formerly St Bartholomew's Hospital, London, UK

Andrew Morgan
Consultant Clinical Scientist, Formerly Head of Radiotherapy Physics, Musgrove Park Hospital, Taunton, UK

Niall MacDougall
Consultant Clinical Scientist, Head of Clinical Dosimetry, Barts Health NHS Trust, UK

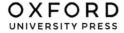

OXFORD
UNIVERSITY PRESS

OXFORD
UNIVERSITY PRESS

Great Clarendon Street, Oxford, OX2 6DP,
United Kingdom

Oxford University Press is a department of the University of Oxford.
It furthers the University's objective of excellence in research, scholarship,
and education by publishing worldwide. Oxford is a registered trade mark of
Oxford University Press in the UK and in certain other countries

© Oxford University Press 2023

The moral rights of the authors have been asserted

First Edition published in 2012
Second Edition published in 2023

Published in the United States of America by Oxford University Press
198 Madison Avenue, New York, NY 10016, United States of America

British Library Cataloguing in Publication Data
Data available

Library of Congress Control Number: 2022943022

ISBN 978-0-19-886286-4

DOI: 10.1093/med/9780198862864.001.0001

Printed and bound by
CPI Group (UK) Ltd, Croydon, CR0 4YY

AS – For Theo, Isabella, James, Naomi, Nuala and Farida
NMD – For Emily and Alistair
AMM – For my ever-patient wife Kàren and for George Pitchford[†] – mentor, colleague, and friend. I have much to thank him for

[†] It is with regret we report the passing of George Pitchford during the preparation of this book.

Contents

† It is with regret we report the passing of George Pitchford during the preparation of this book.

Abbreviations

A	amp	EPR	Environmental Permitting Regulations
AI	artificial intelligence	EQD	equivalent dose
ALARP	as low as reasonably practicable	eV	electron Volts
ARSAC	Administration of Radioactive Substances Advisory Committee	FDG	fluorodeoxyglucose
aSi	amorphous silicon	FFF	flattening filter-free
AV	anti-virus	FOV	field of vision
Ci	curie	FSD	focus-to-surface distance
CPE	charged particle equilibrium	GTV	gross tumour volume
BEV	beam's eye view	GTTV	gross tumour target volume
BIPM	International Bureau of Weights and Measures	Gy	Gray
Bq	Becquerel	HASS	High-Activity Sealed Sources
BSF	backscatter factor	HDR	high dose rate
BSS	Basic Safety Standards	HU	Hounsfield unit
CAP	customer acceptance protocol	HVL	half value layer
CBCT	cone beam computed tomography	Hz	hertz
cGy	centigray	IAEA	International Atomic Energy Authority
CoP	Codes of Practice	ICRU	International Commission on Radiation Units
CQC	Care Quality Commission	IGRT	image-guided radiotherapy
CSDA	continuous slowing down approximation	IM	internal margin
CT	computed tomography	IMPT	intensity modulated proton therapy
CTV	clinical target volume	IMRT	intensity modulated RT
DIBH	deep inspiration breath-hold	IP	Internet Protocol
DICOM	Digital Imaging and Communication in Medicine	IPEM	Institute of Physics and Engineering in Medicine
DoB	date of birth	IR(ME)R	Ionising Radiation (Medical Exposure) Regulations
DoF	degrees of freedom	IRR	Ionising Radiation Regulations
DoH	Department of Health	IT	information technology
DR	dose rate	ITV	internal target volume
DRR	digitally reconstructed radiograph	IVD	*in-vivo* dosimetry
DVH	dose volume histogram	J	joule
EBRT	external beam radiotherapy	kerma	kinetic energy released per unit mass
EC	European Community		
EM	electromagnetic	kV	kilovoltage
EPID	electronic portal imaging device		

kVp	kiloVoltage peak		PTV	planning target volume
LDR	low dose rate		QA	quality assurance
LET	linear energy transfer		QC	quality control
linac	linear accelerator		QI	Quality Index
LMPA	low melting point alloy		QMS	quality management system
LNT	linear no-threshold		R&V	record and verify
mA	milliamperes		RAID	Redundant Array of Independent Discs
MDR	medium dose rate		RAKR	reference air kerma rate
MDT	multidisciplinary team		RBE	relative biological effectiveness
MeV	Mega electron volt		RCR	Royal College of Radiologists
MIRD	medical internal radiation dose		RF	radiofrequency
MLC	multileaf collimator		RPA	radiation protection advisor
MOSFET	metal oxide semiconductor field effect transistor		RPS	radiation protection supervisor
MPE	medical physics expert		RT	radiotherapy
MR	magnetic resonance		RTOG	Radiation Therapy Oncology Group
MRI	magnetic resonance imaging		RTTQA	Radiotherapy Trials Quality Assurance
MRL	magnetic resonance linear		SABR	stereotactic ablative body radiotherapy
MSCC	metastatic spinal cord compression		SAD	source-to-axis distance
mSv	milliSievert		Sc	collimator scatter factor
MU	monitor unit		SCD	source to calibration distance
MV	megavolt/megavoltage		SCF	supraclavicular fossa
NHS	National Health Service		SF	scatter factor
NORM	naturally occurring radioactive materials		SM	setup margin
NPL	National Physical Laboratory		SMR	standardized mortality rate
NRRW	National Registry of Radiation Workers		SOBP	spread out Bragg peak
NTCP	normal tissue complication probability		Sp	phantom scatter factor
OAR	organs at risk		SPECT	single photon emission computed tomography
OD	optical density		SRPD	source to reference point distance
ODI	optical distance indicator		SRS	stereotactic radiosurgery
OF	output factor		SSD	source-to-surface distance
PDD	percentage depth dose		SUV	standardized uptake value
PE	photoelectric		Sv	Sievert
PET	positron emission tomography		SXR	superficial X-rays
POP	parallel opposed pair		TAR	tissue air ratio
PRV	planning organ at risk volume		TBI	total body irradiation
PSDL	primary standard dosimetry laboratory		TCP	tumour control probability
PSF	peak scatter factor		TCPE	transient charged particle equilibrium

TF	transmission factor		TSET	total skin electron therapy
TIFF	tagged image file format		TSRT	Towards Safer Radiotherapy
TL	thermoluminescent		TV	treated volume
TLD	thermoluminescent dosimeter		US	ultrasound
TMR	tissue maximum ratio		V	volt
TPR	tissue phantom ratio		VHEE	very high energy electrons
TPS	treatment planning system		VIBH	voluntary inspiration breath-hold
TRUS	transrectal ultrasound		VMAT	volumetric modulated arc therapy
TSE	total skin electron		WF	wedge factor

Contributors

John Byrne
Newcastle General Hospital,
Newcastle, UK

Susan Corcoran
St Bartholomew's Hospital, London, UK

Christopher Dean
St Bartholomew's Hospital, London, UK

Glenn Flux
Royal Marsden Hospital & Institute of
Cancer Research, Surrey, UK

Jonathan Gear
Royal Marsden Hospital & Institute of
Cancer Research, Surrey, UK

Tony Greener
Guy's and St Thomas's Hospital,
London, UK

Alan Hounsell
Northern Ireland Cancer Centre, Belfast
City Hospital, Northern Ireland

Frances Lavender
Royal Marsden Hospital, London, UK

Niall MacDougall
St Bartholomews Hospital, London, UK

Ranald Mackay
Christie Hospital, Manchester, UK

Andrew Morgan
Musgrove Park Hospital, Taunton, UK

Andrew Nisbet
University College London, London, UK

George Pitchford[†]
Formerly United Lincolnshire NHS
Hospitals Trust
Lincoln, UK

Brenda Pratt
Royal Marsden Hospital & Institute of
Cancer Research, Surrey, UK

Ondrée Severn
St Bartholomew's Hospital,
London, UK

Amen Sibtain
St Bartholomew's Hospital, London, UK

Jim Thurston
Dorset County Hospital, Dorchester, UK

Gemma Whitelaw
St Bartholomew's Hospital,
London, UK

[†] It is with regret we report the passing of George Pitchford during the preparation of this book.

Introduction

'*Everything should be made as simple as possible, but no simpler*'
Quotation attributed to Albert Einstein (1933)

We are delighted to have produced this second edition of *Physics for Clinical Oncology*, twelve years after we first conceived the project with Oxford University Press. Whilst the fundamentals have not changed, advances in technology have driven the need for an update. We are grateful that the first edition was very positively received but we have also listened carefully to feedback. We have made every effort to improve on the work by refreshing and updating each chapter thoroughly but we still aim to take the clinical oncologist through the essentials of radiotherapy physics in a relatively concise format through including important detail with an explanatory style.

The successful structure of the text has been maintained using the Royal College of Radiologists syllabus for radiotherapy physics as a guide. We begin by explaining the absolute basics in the first three chapters, followed by chapters on more advanced topics to give a comprehensive understanding of physics in radiotherapy.

The authors again have been chosen for their expertise and talent for explaining complex topics with clarity and concision. We thank all of them from both editions for devoting their time, effort, and skill for this book. We also are grateful to the team at Oxford University Press, in particular Janine Fisher and Caroline Smith for their constant support and patience.

We hope the book serves its purpose supporting trainees in all areas of radiotherapy.

Amen Sibtain
Andrew Morgan
Niall MacDougall

Chapter 1

Basic physics essentials to the radiation oncologist

Amen Sibtain, Andrew Morgan, and Niall MacDougall

1.1 The absolute basics

1.1.1 Elements and compounds

Everything is made up of matter. There are two types of matter—elements and compounds.

1.1.1.1 Traditional definition of an element

An element is a kind of matter that **cannot** be decomposed into more than two simpler types of matter. An example of an element is hydrogen.

1.1.1.2 Definition of a compound

A compound is a kind of matter that **can** be decomposed into more than two simpler types of matter.

1.1.1.3 An alternative definition of a compound

A compound is formed when two or more elements combine to produce a more complex kind of matter. An example of a compound is water, which can be broken down into the two elements, hydrogen and oxygen.

1.2 Atoms and molecules

Atoms are the very smallest particles of an element that can exist without losing the chemical properties of that element. There are 118 types of atom, all defined in the periodic table by their atomic numbers. The periodic table arranges the atoms in groups and in periods. The rows are called periods and the columns are called groups. Elements in the same group are similar to each other.

Molecules are the smallest particles of a compound that can exist without losing the chemical properties of that compound—for example, the water molecule consisting of two hydrogen atoms and one oxygen atom. If the molecule is broken down further the resulting matter loses the properties of water.

1.2.1 **Atomic substructure**

Atoms can be broken down into smaller particles. These particles are neutrons, protons, and electrons.

Neutrons and protons are in the nucleus of the atom and are surrounded by the electrons.

Protons are relatively large particles and have a positive charge. Neutrons are also 'large' but have no charge (see Table 1.1).

Electrons are relatively much smaller and lighter particles. They are attracted to the nucleus because they have a negative charge, but they do not collide with it because the electrons orbit the nucleus.

It is easy to imagine the atom as a group of billiard balls in the nucleus with smaller balls—the electrons—moving around the nucleus in the same way the planets of the solar system orbit the sun—so a hydrogen atom with one proton in the nucleus and one orbiting electron would look like that in Figure 1.1.

There are two things wrong with this way of imagining atoms. First, the electron is actually much further away from the nucleus than the figure depicts—if it were drawn to scale it would be about 500 metres away. An atom is therefore mostly space. Second, whilst protons and neutrons do behave as particles, electrons also have wave-type behaviour, like light. Rather than moving in a fixed path around the nucleus like a 'planet', there is a cloud of electron waves around the nucleus. The wave/particle paradox has been thoroughly explored over the past century. However, for the purposes of radiotherapy, electrons should be imagined as particles.

1.2.2 **Atomic and mass numbers**

Each atom has a particular number of protons and neutrons.

The mass number, A, of an atom is the number of the protons and neutrons added together. The symbol A is from the German word *Atomgewicht*, meaning atomic weight.

The atomic number, Z, is the number of protons in the nucleus, this comes from the German word *Zahl*, meaning number.

The atomic and mass numbers are depicted as:

$$_{Z}^{A} X$$

Table 1.1 The charge and mass of subatomic particles

Name	Charge	Mass
Proton	positive	1.6726×10^{-27} kg
Neutron	neutral	1.6929×10^{-27} kg
Electron	negative	9.11×10^{-31} kg

Charge is measured in Coulombs (C). The absolute value of charge of a proton and an electron is 1.602×10^{-19} C.

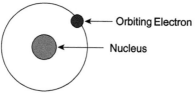

Figure 1.1 A hydrogen atom.

The atomic number defines the atom and hence the element. If the number of protons is somehow changed, the atom changes into that of another element. In contrast, if the number of neutrons is changed, the atom remains the same, but it may have some different characteristics. Atoms with the same atomic number but different mass numbers are called **isotopes**.

1.3 Electron shells and energy levels

1.3.1 Electron shells

Electrons reside around the nucleus in a number of 'shells' (Figure 1.2). They cannot exist between these shells.

The shells are labelled with letters of the alphabet, starting with K at the inner shell. Each shell can hold a maximum number of electrons.

Every shell, apart from the K-shell, is made up of sub-shells.

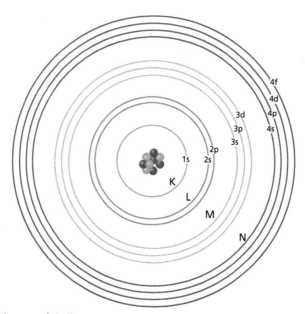

Figure 1.2 Diagram of shells.

Table 1.2 Atomic electron shells and sub-shells with their electron capacity

Shell	Maximum electron capacity	Sub-shells	Maximum sub-shell electron capacity
K	2	1s	2
L	8	2s	2
		2p	6
M	18	3s	2
		3p	6
		3d	10
N	32	4s	2
		4p	6
		4d	10
		4f	14
O	50	5s	2
		5p	6
		5d	10
		5f	14
		5g	18

The shell closest to the nucleus (K) has one sub-shell, which can hold a maximum of two electrons. The next shell out (L) has two sub-shells—one holding a maximum of two and the second capable of holding a maximum of six electrons. The next shell (M) has 3 sub-shells, holding two, six, and ten electrons respectively. This is summarized in Table 1.2.

1.3.2 Binding energy

The electrons are held in their shell by their electrostatic attraction to the positively charged nucleus. To remove an electron from a shell, a certain amount of energy is needed to overcome this attraction. This is called the **binding energy** (Figure 1.3). The binding energy is greatest for the inner shell and is progressively lower for each shell moving away from the nucleus. Binding energies are greater for atoms with a greater number of protons in the nucleus (i.e. a higher atomic number) because they have a higher positive nuclear charge, and therefore have a greater hold on the orbiting electrons. Binding energies are usually quoted in electron Volts (eV). 1 eV is defined as the energy obtained by one electron accelerated across 1 Volt, 1 eV = 1.602 $\times$ 10^{-19} Joules.

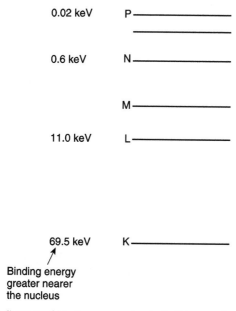

Figure 1.3 Example diagram of binding energy levels, in this case, for tungsten.

If an electron gains more energy than the binding energy, it can escape from the attraction of the nucleus and leave the atom. This is called **ionization**. The resulting atom has a net positive charge because it has one less electron than it has protons—that is, it is a positive ion.

1.3.3 Energy levels

An electron can also move between shells of different binding energies. This happens when an electron gains enough energy to move from one (sub-) shell to another, but not quite enough to escape the atom completely. Each (sub-) shell can therefore be thought of as a fixed energy level and electrons can only exist in these shells if they possess that particular amount of energy. The energy levels are fixed for any particular type of atom (Figure 1.4).

As well as moving from a lower energy level to a higher energy level by gaining energy from somewhere, electrons can move the other way and release their excess energy.

1.3.4 Energy levels for isolated atoms and interacting atoms

The energy levels are exact for isolated atoms. However, when a number of atoms are together, such as in a molecule or as a solid element, the electron shells interact. This interaction allows each fixed energy level to expand to a range, which is called an energy band (Figure 1.5).

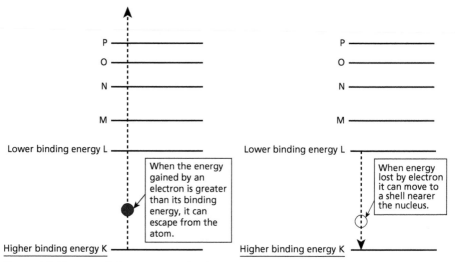

Figure 1.4 Diagram of electron energy level movement.

1.4 **Electromagnetism, electromagnetic radiation, and the electromagnetic spectrum**

1.4.1 **The four fundamental forces of nature**

The forces of nature are:

- gravity
- electromagnetism
- weak interaction
- strong interaction

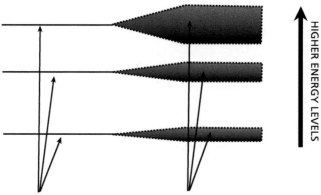

Figure 1.5 Diagram of energy bands within solids.

They are termed 'fundamental' because they cannot be explained or picked apart by other forces. They form the basis of all interactions in nature. Several theories exist to understand and unify these fundamental forces but these are beyond the scope of this book and not needed to understand radiotherapy physics. Gravity is not relevant to atomic interactions and the strong and weak interactions are discussed in section 1.5.1.

1.4.2 Electromagnetism

Electromagnetism is one of these fundamental forces and it describes the force of a magnetic field on a moving charged particle. Similarly, it describes how moving charged particles create magnetic fields.

1.4.3 Electromagnetic radiation

Electromagnetic radiation is a form of energy transfer though space as a combination of electrical and magnetic fields. A moving electrical field generates a varying magnetic field and vice versa. These combined moving fields form the electromagnetic wave. An unusual feature of electromagnetic radiation is that it sometimes behaves as waves and sometimes behaves as particles—summed up in the term 'wave-particle duality'.

1.4.3.1 The wave model of electromagnetic radiation

Electromagnetic radiation causes effects that suggest it behaves as waves. For example, it exhibits reflection, refraction, and interference. All electromagnetic waves travel at a velocity of 3×10^8 metres per second in a vacuum.

1.4.4 Waves

Waves are a series of peaks and troughs and have definable features: wavelength, frequency, and energy (Figure 1.6).

Wavelength is the distance between two successive crests or troughs. The symbol for wavelength is λ and it is measured in metres.

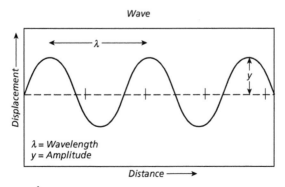

Figure 1.6 Diagram of a wave.

Frequency is the number of waves passing a particular point per unit time. The symbol is v and the unit is number per second or hertz (Hz).

The amplitude can be thought of as the energy of the wave.

1.4.5 The particle behaviour of electromagnetic radiation

Electromagnetic radiation also behaves as particles. These particles are discrete packets of energy called photons. The energy of these photons is proportional to the frequency of the electromagnetic wave to which they are linked. There is an equation that relates the energy and frequency called the Planck–Einstein equation:

$$E = h.v$$

where E is energy, h is Planck's constant (6.626×10^{-34} J/s) and v is frequency. So if frequency is the velocity divided by the wavelength, then

$$E = h.c/\lambda$$

where c is the speed of light and λ is the wavelength of the wave.

Given h and c are constant, wavelength and energy are inversely proportional to each other; that is, a short wavelength relates to high energy photons and a long wavelength to low energy photons. We can also say frequency and wavelength vary together. At high frequencies and short wavelengths, and therefore higher energies, electromagnetic radiation has more particle-like behaviour.

The range of frequency and wavelengths is called the electromagnetic spectrum (Figure 1.7). Humans have evolved to detect part of this spectrum—visible light. The rest of the electromagnetic spectrum on either side of visible light cannot be sensed. X-rays/gamma rays are in the high frequency, short wavelength (high energy) part of this spectrum. There is no hard boundary between X-rays and gamma rays but it may be useful to remember that X-rays are electronic in origin and gamma rays are nuclear in origin.

1.5 Radioactivity

1.5.1 Summary of atomic structure

Atoms consist of a central nucleus surrounded by an electron cloud. The nucleus is made up of neutrons and protons, held together by a strong force, called the 'strong nuclear force' to make it easy to remember! The strong nuclear force is one of the fundamental forces of nature. The weak nuclear force is responsible for radioactive decay, and the electrostatic force is involved in holding electrons around the nucleus.

1.5.2 The essence of radioactivity

Sub-atomic particles exist in a particular arrangement. The amount of energy in the particles can vary with the arrangement. They will always try to settle in an

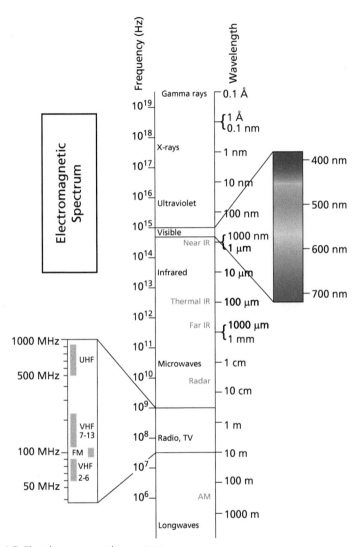

Figure 1.7 The electromagnetic spectrum.

arrangement that has the lowest energy configuration. Some nuclides have unstable nuclear arrangements and shift to a more stable arrangement over time. While undergoing this arrangement they emit one of the following:

♦ an alpha particle: a particle consisting of two protons and two neutrons

♦ a beta particle: a negatively charged electron or positively charged positron

♦ a gamma ray: a packet of electromagnetic energy, that is, a photon.

Any element that undergoes this process is called 'radioactive', and the phenomenon is called 'radioactivity'.

Another way of regarding radioactive materials is that they continuously emit energy in the form of the alpha particles, beta particles or electromagnetic waves.

1.5.3 The decay series: parent and daughter

Radioactive materials undergo a series of transformations until they reach a stable state. These transformations occur in a series of steps. These steps are called the 'decay series'. The original element is called the 'parent' and the stable 'end-result' element is the 'stable daughter' (Figure 1.8). The isotopes or elements in between are the 'excited daughter'.

1.5.4 Types of radioactive decay in more detail

1.5.4.1 Alpha decay

Alpha decay is the emission of alpha particles by a nucleus. Alpha particles are denoted by the symbol α.

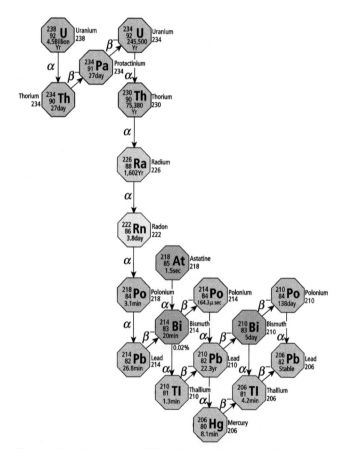

Figure 1.8 The uranium decay series, U238 being the 'parent' and lead 206 being the stable daughter. All other elements in the series are the 'excited daughters'.

Alpha particles are made up of 2 neutrons and 2 protons. They have a charge of +2 because each proton has a positive charge and neutrons have no charge. They are slow moving and relatively heavy particles. They can be deflected in a magnetic field and can be stopped easily by a sheet of paper. They can cause significant damage to body tissue if ingested. Only larger nuclei, where Z exceeds 82, undergo alpha decay. It results in the formation of a new element because of the loss of protons.

When an atom loses an alpha particle, the atomic number reduces by 2 (i.e. the number of protons that are lost) and the mass number reduces by 4 (i.e. the number of protons plus the number of neutrons that are lost).

For example, radium has a mass number of 226 and an atomic number of 88. It undergoes alpha decay, losing 2 protons and 2 neutrons, and becomes radon, which has a mass number of 222 and an atomic number of 86.

$$^{226}_{88}Ra \rightarrow\ ^{222}_{86}Rn + {}^{4}_{2}\alpha$$

It should be noted that when writing about isotopes, they can be referred to in the form 'isotope name-atomic mass', for example radium-226.

1.5.4.2 Beta decay

Beta particles can carry either a positive charge or a negative charge. Those with a negative charge are electrons, indicated by e⁻ and those with a positive charge are called positrons, indicated by e⁺.

The emission of a negative beta particle, that is an electron, is called *beta minus decay* and the emission of a positive beta particle is called *beta positive decay*.

1.5.4.3 Beta minus decay

Beta minus decay occurs when a neutron in the nucleus converts into a proton and an electron. The electrons can travel a few metres in air but are easily stopped by a thin sheet of aluminium or glass. The electron (known as e⁻ or β⁻) is emitted along with another particle called an anti-neutrino. Neutrinos and anti-neutrinos are small particles with zero mass. They are of great interest to particle physicists but are of no relevance in radiotherapy.

This conversion means the mass number stays the same that is, the loss of the neutron is offset by the gain of a proton. However, the atomic number increases by 1, that is the net gain of that proton.

The electron/beta particle is released with a certain amount of kinetic energy. The maximum possible kinetic energy is equal to the difference in the mass between the original nucleus and the post-emission nucleus. Not all beta particles carry the maximum possible amount of kinetic energy; it is usually less than that. The remaining energy released is carried by the antineutrino. So caesium-137 decays to barium-137m as:

$$^{137}_{55}Cs \rightarrow\ ^{137m}_{56}Ba + e^- + antineutrino$$

Note that the 'm' denotes that the barium nucleus is 'metastable', meaning that it still has excess energy to lose. This is often by the emission of a gamma ray.

If a nucleus decays to a lower energy state without changing its number of protons or neutrons it is said to be an isomer. It is actually the gamma decay of barium-137m that produces the photon that gives caesium-137 its therapeutic properties.

1.5.4.4 Beta positive decay

Beta positive decay occurs when a proton in the nucleus is converted into a neutron and a positron. The positron (known as e⁺ or β⁺) is emitted along with another particle called a neutrino. The atomic number reduces by one due to a net loss of protons, but again, the mass number remains the same because the total number of protons and neutrons does not change.

Positrons, once released, lose their kinetic energy in the same way as electrons do. When most of this has gone, the positron combines with an electron. Their combined mass turns into two 511 keV photons, each traveling in opposite directions from the point of the annihilation.

This is the key process underlying Positron Emission Tomography (PET) imaging where fluorine-18 decays to oxygen-18, emitting a positron and a neutrino.

$$^{18}_{9}F \rightarrow {}^{18}_{8}O + e^{+} + \text{neutrino}$$

1.5.4.5 Electron capture

In electron capture, the nucleus combines with one of the orbiting electrons, converting one of its protons into a neutron, and releasing a neutrino. Usually a K-shell electron is captured. The atomic number decreases by one because there is one less proton. The mass number remains the same because the number of protons plus neutrons has not changed.

The loss of an electron in the K-shell leaves the atom energetically unstable and so an electron from a higher orbital fills the vacancy in the K-shell. The electron that fills the vacancy is, by definition, losing energy. This excess energy is released as photons or electrons. Electrons emitted in this way are called Auger electrons (Figure 1.9).

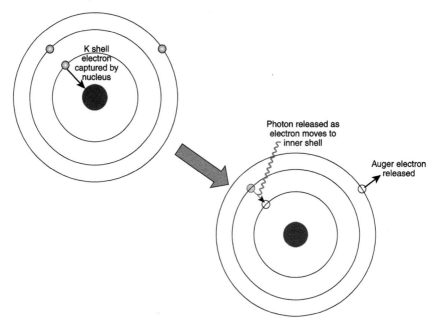

Figure 1.9 Electron capture producing Auger electrons.

An example of electron capture is:

$$_{53}^{125}I + K \, shell \, e^- \rightarrow _{52}^{125}Te + neutrino$$

1.5.4.6 Gamma rays

These are packets of electromagnetic rays that originate from the nucleus. Beta-positive and beta-negative decay often leave the nucleus energetically unstable, and this excess energy is released as gamma rays. Extremely high energy gamma rays can penetrate several metres of dense material such as concrete.

For example, Cobalt 60

$$_{27}^{60}Co \rightarrow _{28}^{60}Ni + e^- + antineutrino$$

$$_{28}^{60}Ni \rightarrow _{28}^{60}Ni + 1.17 \, MeV \, gamma + 1.3 \, MeV \, gamma$$

1.5.4.7 Internal conversion

In contrast to gamma decay, where an energetic nucleus releases its excess energy as a photon, the energy can be transferred to an orbiting electron, usually a K-shell electron. The electron then uses some of this energy to escape the atom, and travels with what is left of the energy, as kinetic energy.

The resulting vacancy is filled by an electron from a higher energy level. The cascade of electrons to the lowest overall energy state releases the excess energy as photons or Auger electrons.

1.5.5 Activity and half-life

The activity of a radioactive material is measured as the number of atoms that disintegrate per second. The SI unit of activity is the **becquerel**, the symbol is **Bq**. The unit is named after Antoine Henri Becquerel, a French physicist who won the Nobel Prize in Physics in 1903 as the discoverer of radioactivity. One of his doctoral students was Marie Curie, after whom another unit of radioactivity, the **curie** (symbol **Ci**) is named. One curie is approximately the activity of 1 gram of radium 226, which decays at the rate of 3.7×10^{10} disintegrations per second: $1 \, Ci = 3.7 \times 10^{10}$ Bq.

The activity of any radioactive material reduces with time. The activity at any particular time is dependent on the number of atoms present at that time. The proportion of atoms undergoing disintegration remains constant. This leads to a pattern of decay called 'exponential decay'.

Half-life is defined as the time for a radioactive material to lose half of its activity, which is the same as saying it is the time for half the atoms in a material to decay (Figure 1.10).

The mathematical equation describing the activity at any particular time is:

$$A_t = A_o e^{-\lambda t}$$

A_t is the activity at the time, t

A_o is the activity at time zero

λ is a constant which depends on the half-life $T_{1/2}$

$\lambda = 0.6931/T_{1/2}$

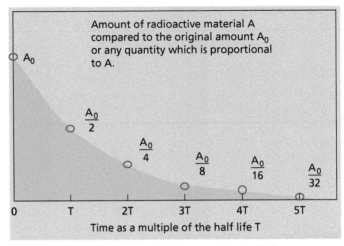

Figure 1.10 A graph illustrating exponential decay and the half-life.

1.5.5.1 Sources of radioactive materials

Radioactive materials are either naturally occurring or artificially produced.

1.5.5.2 Naturally occurring radioactive materials

There are three naturally occurring radioactive decay series:

Uranium-238 ---------> (Radium-226) ----------> Lead-206

Actinium-235 ---> Lead-207

Thorium-232 ---> Lead-208

These naturally occurring radioactive materials tend to have high atomic numbers. The half-life is longer for those with a higher atomic number. They all decay to lead (Figure 1.8) and undergo a series of steps in this decay. For example, uranium, with a half-life of 4.5 billion years, emits an alpha particle to become thorium-234, which in turn emits a beta particle to become protactinium-234, and a further 11 steps to become lead-206.

Whilst radium was the first radioactive isotope used for therapy, this small family of isotopes are not considered safe: they have a long half-life and emit gas and decay by emission of alpha particles. However, radium-223 which has a short half-life of 11.4 days is now widely used as an unsealed source in the treatment of metastatic bone disease.

1.5.6 Artificially produced radioactive materials

Artificially produced radioactive materials are made in one of three ways:

1) Fission

2) Neutron bombardment

3) Charged particle bombardment

1.5.6.1 Fission

Fission occurs in a nuclear reactor. It is the splitting of a large atom into roughly two equal parts. It occurs when a neutron (denoted by $_0^1 n$) enters a nucleus, making the nucleus unstable and leads to new atoms resulting from the fusion of one or more neutrons that have kinetic energy, and energy in the form of neutrinos and gamma rays.

In nuclear fission, uranium-235 splits into two separate atoms, one or more neutrons and a lot of energy. There are many possible products of nuclear fission, one example being:

$$^{235}_{92}U + ^{1}_{0}n \rightarrow ^{134}_{54}Xe + ^{100}_{38}Sr + ^{1}_{0}n + ^{1}_{0}n + energy$$

The neutrons then react with other uranium nuclei and the reaction continues as a chain reaction.

Fission reactions can produce:

Strontium-90, used for the treatment of ocular tumours

Caesium-137, formerly used in moderate dose rate brachytherapy

1.5.6.2 Neutron bombardment

Here, a stable element is placed in a nuclear reactor and bombarded with neutrons. The nucleus of the stable element captures a neutron. This leads to rearrangement of the nuclear components and the release of energy in the form of gamma rays.

Cobalt-60, used in many external beam therapy machines around the world, is produced in this way. Other useful products of neutron bombardment are phosphorus-32, previously used in the treatment of polycythaemia, molybdenum-99 that decays to the metastable isomer, technetium-99m which is used for bone scans, and tellurium-131 which decays to iodine-131, used in imaging and treatment of thyroid disease.

1.5.6.3 Charged particle bombardment

This is when a stable element is bombarded with protons or alpha particles using a cyclotron leading to absorption of the particle and ejection of one or more neutrons. The resulting element has a higher atomic number, that is, a proton gain. Fluorine-19 is produced in this way, used in the PET imaging of malignant disease.

Chapter 2

The life of a photon: Birth to extinction and what happens in between

Amen Sibtain, Andrew Morgan, and Niall MacDougall

2.1 In the beginning

X-rays were discovered by Wilhelm Conrad Roentgen in the late afternoon of 8 November 1895. Within two weeks he had taken an X-ray image of his wife's hand, and by the end of the year he published the paper, 'On A New Kind of Rays' ('*Über eine neue Art von Strahlen*'). The discovery earned him the Nobel Prize in 1901, around the time of the discovery of radium. He called them X-rays because he didn't know what they were; in algebra, X denotes an unknown, so he called them X-rays, and the name stuck.

2.2 The birth of a photon: X-ray production

X-rays are electromagnetic radiation at the 'high-energy end' of the electromagnetic spectrum (Figure 1.7). They are formed when electrons travelling at high velocity interact with other electrons or nuclei in matter that has a high atomic number. These interactions can be collisions or close encounters. The electron loses energy from these interactions, and this energy is released as electromagnetic waves: **the photon is born!**

There are a range of possible interactions the travelling electron can have:

1) Interactions with orbiting electrons, either
   (a) Outer orbiting electrons
   (b) Inner orbiting electrons
2) Interactions with the nucleus
3) Collisions with the nucleus

2.2.1 Interactions with the orbiting electrons

2.2.1.1 Outer orbiting electrons

The travelling electron can impart energy to an orbiting electron which can gain enough energy to escape from the nucleus it is orbiting along with any excess energy. This interaction is called **ionization**; a photon is **not** produced.

The amount of energy delivered may be not enough to cause ionization but only enough to cause the electron to vibrate. The travelling electron continues on its journey, with less kinetic energy and in a different direction.

2.2.1.2 Inner orbiting electrons

The travelling electron interacts with an inner shell electron (either a K- or L-shell, section 1.3.1). The energy transferred allows the inner shell electron to escape the atom, ie ionization. The vacancy in the K- or L-shell is filled by an electron from an M- or N-shell. The electrons in the more distant shells have a higher energy. When dropping to a lower energy level they release their excess energy as electromagnetic radiation, i.e. photons. The energy released is the difference between the binding energy of the two shells the electron moved between which is different for each atom. These are characteristic X-rays.

2.2.2 Characteristic X-rays

The electron shells in a particular atom have their own particular binding energy. The binding energy of each shell depends on the atomic number of that particular element, i.e the mass of the nucleus. The larger the nucleus is, the more protons there are, so the greater the binding energy of the electron shells. Therefore, when an inner shell electron is removed from any particular atom and a higher shell electron fills that vacancy, the energy of the resulting photon is also particular to that element. The range of photon energies that emanate from that element are the **characteristic X-rays** of that element.

2.2.3 Interactions with the nucleus

The nucleus carries a positive charge and the electron carries a negative charge. The nucleus is also substantially larger than the electron. A passing electron travelling at high speed near a nucleus will be influenced by this attraction and, as a result, will change direction and lose some of its kinetic energy. This 'lost energy' is released as electromagnetic energy, a photon. The electron will slow down, as though it has 'put the brakes on'. The photons/X-rays/electromagnetic radiation (all the same thing) released in this way are called 'braking radiation', more usually using the German, '*bremsstrahlung*'.

This mechanism of X-ray production produces a wide range of energies across the X-ray spectrum, ranging from very low to up to that of the maximum kinetic energy of the incoming electrons.

Bremsstrahlung is the dominant way in which clinical X-rays are produced when high atomic number materials are irradiated with electrons.

2.2.4 Collisions with the nucleus

This is a rare event for electrons and not relevant to radiotherapy.

2.3 The basic components of an X-ray tube: how to bring photons to life

To bring photons to life we need an instrument that can:

♦ generate electrons

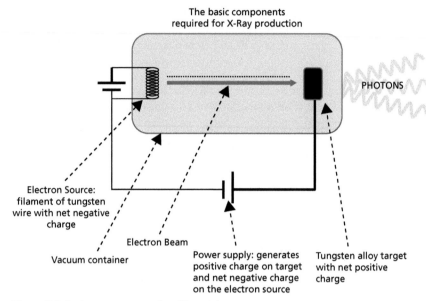

The basic components
required for X-Ray production

PHOTONS

Electron Source:
filament of tungsten
wire with net negative
charge

Vacuum container

Electron Beam

Power supply: generates
positive charge on target
and net negative charge
on the electron source

Tungsten alloy target
with net positive
charge

Figure 2.1 Basic components of an X-ray tube.

♦ move these electrons at high speed (i.e. give them kinetic energy)
♦ direct them at a high atomic number target

The basic components of this instrument—the X-ray tube (Figure 2.1)—are therefore:

♦ an electron source to generate the electrons
♦ a positively charged target in which the electrons can interact
♦ a vacuum container to give the electrons a clear path to the target
♦ a high voltage power supply

2.3.1 **The electron source**

This is a thin filament of tungsten wire that has a high electrical current passed through it; in other words, there are lots of electrons flowing through the wire. The current/ number of electrons is so high that the filament heats up and some electrons escape the wire and form a cloud of electrons around it.

The filament current can be varied which in turn varies the number of electrons emitted into the electron cloud. The higher the current, the hotter the filament gets, and the more electrons are emitted. This process is described in section 11.2.2 for radiotherapy equipment.

2.3.2 **The target**

The target needs to contain a high atomic number material to give plenty of opportunity for bremsstrahlung to occur. It also needs a high melting point and to be able to conduct heat away effectively. It is therefore made of a tungsten alloy.

2.3.3 **The power supply**

The power supply generates the positive charge on the target. The higher the voltage in the system the greater the difference in charge between the negatively charged electron source (the cathode) and the positively charged target (anode).

These basic components are similar for all X-ray machines, from diagnostic to low energy therapy. The details of a linear accelerator are given in section 11.4.

2.3.4 **The X-ray spectrum**

When X-rays are produced by electrons entering a target, a range of photon energies results. If drawn as a histogram with the energy value on the x-axis and the frequency of each energy on the y-axis, the result is as in Figure 2.2.

The vertical axis is also referred to as the 'intensity', which basically refers to the amount of radiation produced at any given energy. Note that when referring to a specific photon energy, the term keV is used but when talking about an X-ray spectrum, the term kVp (kiloVoltage peak) is used. So a photon beam generated using an electron beam with an energy of 150 keV would be referred to as a 150 kVp beam.

There are two parts to the X-ray spectrum.

1) There is a *continuous spectrum* that results from bremsstrahlung. The continuous spectrum depends on the energy of the incoming electrons and is the same for any target material.

2) There are narrow spikes of particular energy intensities that are due to atomic properties of the target material, which are the *characteristic* X-ray part of the spectrum.

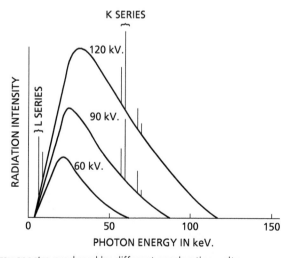

Figure 2.2 X-ray spectra produced by different accelerating voltages.
Reproduced with permission from Meredith and Massey, *The Fundamental Physics of Radiology*, 3rd Edition, J Wright, 1977.

Note that, despite the appearance of the graph above, very low energy photons will be produced by the target; these will be absorbed in the walls of the X-ray tube and cannot be measured directly.

2.3.5 Adjusting the intensity and quality of the X-rays

2.3.5.1 Radiation intensity

The radiation intensity depends linearly on three parameters:

1) the atomic number Z of the target material
2) the square of the accelerating potential of the tube (kV²)
3) the current of the beam, that is the number of electrons crossing the tube

Obviously once a tube has been produced, the atomic number of the target is fixed, but for different tubes with different targets, the intensity will vary linearly as the atomic number changes.

Increasing the intensity of radiation being produced in a particular time requires an increase in the number of electrons being produced—more electrons will produce more photons.

2.3.5.2 X-ray beam quality

The *quality* of an X-ray beam describes its penetrating power. It depends on the energy of the photons in the beam and therefore depends on the energy of the electrons entering the target. The quality of the beam is therefore increased by increasing the tube voltage.

2.3.6 Which way do the photons travel?

The direction newly formed photons travel after production is discussed in more detail in section 11.2.1. Referring to Figure 11.1, at low kilovoltage (kV) energies (approximately 100 kVp), the photons produced travel more or less in all directions, i.e. isotropically. As the energy of the electron beam increases, the direction of photon travel starts to bias towards the direction of travel of the original electron beam—the 'forward direction'. In the megavoltage energy range, most photons are produced in the forward direction. This phenomenon influences the design of targets used in therapy equipment. At low kilo-voltage energies, the photon beam emerges isotropically to the electron beam but at megavoltage energy is the photon beam emerges from the target in the same direction as the electron beam.

2.4 Photon interaction with matter: the beginning of the end

The photon interactions described earlier discuss the interaction at an atomic/single photon level. However, a photon beam is a continuous stream of photons. The interaction of the beam with matter is the focus of this section.

When a photon beam leaves a radiation source it has a particular intensity, called **fluence**. The fluence is the number of photons passing through a sphere of unit area in space per unit time. The greater the fluence, the greater the number of photons. The energy fluence is the total energy carried by these photons as a whole.

The intensity of a beam reduces as it passes through a material. This reduction in intensity is called attenuation.

There are two processes at play in photon beam attenuation:

1) Absorption—when a photon gives up all its energy to the material by transferring it to an electron

2) Scatter—the photon collides with an electron or atom and changes direction with or without a change in energy

When a photon enters matter, there are three processes that can occur. Which one of these occurs depends on the energy of the incident photon and the matter with which the photon is interacting.

The interactions are called:

♦ Photoelectric interaction

♦ Compton scatter

♦ Pair production

These interactions all compete with each other, but the probability of any one of them happening depends on, to varying degrees:

♦ the energy of the photon

♦ the atomic number (Z) of the material

2.4.1 Photoelectric interaction

Photoelectric interaction is similar to the 'inner electron interaction' that occurs when an electron interacts with an atom's inner shell electron, described earlier. The difference here is that it is a photon, rather than an electron, that gives up all its energy to an inner shell bound electron. The energy given to the electron can allow it to escape the binding energy of the nucleus, and the vacancy is filled with an electron from another, higher energy shell (Figure 2.3). The energy released by the electron filling the vacancy is released as a photon, which carries energy equal to the difference in the binding energies between the two shells it travels between. *This energy is the characteristic radiation of the material: characteristic X-rays.*

The K-shell characteristic X-ray energies vary from material to material:

Carbon	0.3 keV
Oxygen	0.5 keV
Calcium	4 keV
Lead	88 keV

The probability of photoelectric interaction is:

♦ Directly proportional to the atomic number cubed (Z^3)

♦ Inversely proportional to the energy of the photon cubed (E^{-3})

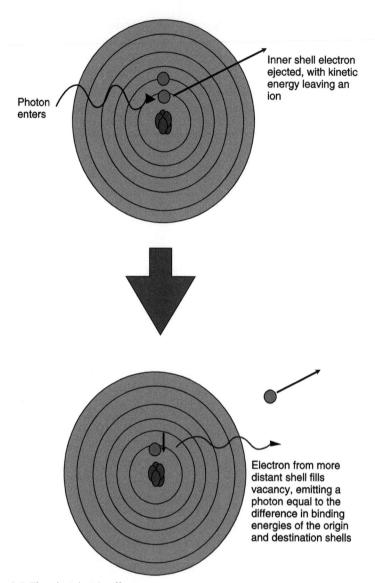

Photon
enters

Inner shell electron
ejected, with kinetic
energy leaving an
ion

Electron from more
distant shell fills
vacancy, emitting a
photon equal to the
difference in binding
energies of the origin
and destination shells

Figure 2.3 The photelectric effect.

Therefore, photoelectric interaction probability increases very rapidly as the atomic number of the material increases and the energy of the photons decrease.

So with low energy photons the photoelectric effect is predominant; this interaction leads to most of the energy of the incoming photons being absorbed.

Practically, the photoelectric effect is most relevant in diagnostic radiology, leading to high contrast between tissues of different densities and atomic numbers—those with higher density and atomic numbers such as bone, containing calcium, are more likely to interact with the incoming low energy photon, absorbing its energy, compared to soft tissue which is predominantly made up of water.

2.4.2 Compton interaction

Compton interaction, also called Compton scattering, is named after the US physicist, Arthur H Compton. **It is the most relevant interaction that occurs in the photon energies used in radiation therapy.**

It can be thought of as a snooker ball like interaction. A travelling photon collides with an electron. *Some* of the photon's energy is transferred to the electron. The electron then moves off with this energy. The photon continues on with less energy, but in a different direction. The greater the angle by which the photon's direction changes, the greater the energy transferred between the photon and the electron.

The angle at which the photon direction changes can range from very slight 'glancing blow' to 180 degrees—a head-on collision. The electron moves off at any angle between 0 and +/–90 degrees. Increasing the photon energy results in the photons being scattered more in the forward direction, as the 'glancing blow' is more likely.

Figures 2.4 and 2.5 show how the angular distribution of the scattered photon and the scattered electron varies with different initial photon energies.

The probability of Compton interaction:

◆ decreases with increasing photon energy in the megavoltage (MV) range (decreases as E^{-1})

◆ is independent of the atomic number of the material with which the photon is interacting

2.4.2.1 Elastic and inelastic scattering

Compton scatter/interaction is also called **inelastic scattering** because energy of the incoming photon is reduced. The original photon energy is redistributed between itself and the electron it interacts with, though the overall energy is conserved.

Elastic (also called Rayleigh) scattering occurs when a photon interacts with a bound atomic electron but does not have enough energy to free it from the atom. This occurs

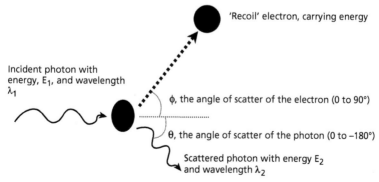

Incident photon with energy, E_1, and wavelength λ_1

'Recoil' electron, carrying energy

ϕ, the angle of scatter of the electron (0 to 90°)

θ, the angle of scatter of the photon (0 to –180°)

Scattered photon with energy E_2 and wavelength λ_2

Figure 2.4 Compton scatter.

$$\lambda_2 - \lambda_1 = \Delta\lambda = \left(\frac{h}{mc}\right)(1 - \cos\theta)$$

λ_1 The wavelength of the incident photon

λ_2 The wavelength of the scattered photon

h   Planck's constant

m   The mass of an electron

c   The speed of light

$\cos\theta$ The cosine of the angle of scatter of the photon

The difference in wavelength, $\Delta\lambda$, between the incident and the scattered photon describes the energy given to the electron. This difference is a maximum when $\theta = 180$ degrees, so the energy transferred to the electron is a maximum when the photon bounces straight back along its original direction of travel.

Figure 2.5 An explanation of the Compton equation.

only when the photon energy is very low. The net effect is that the material takes up no energy and the photon just changes direction. Elastic scattering is an irrelevant effect in radiotherapy.

2.4.3 **Pair production**

This occurs when a photon passes close to a nucleus and changes from a packet of electromagnetic wave energy into a pair of particles—an electron and a positron. All the energy carried by the incoming photon is converted to the mass and kinetic energy of these particles.

The pair of particles then deposits their energy in the material. The positron interacts with an electron and the mass of the two combining particles turns into two photons. The energy of these photons is 0.511 MeV each. This means pair production can only occur if the energy of the incoming photon at the start of the process is greater than 1.022 MeV (the combined energy of the electron and positron created).

The probability of pair production is:

- directly proportional to the atomic number, Z, of the material
- directly proportional to the energy of the photon, E

2.4.4 **Photo-nuclear interactions**

If a photon with energy higher than 8 MeV is absorbed by a nucleus, a neutron can be ejected, in a process called a photo-nuclear interaction. This interaction mainly takes place with heavy nuclei, such as the heavy metals in the head of the treatment machine (tungsten and lead) only at clinical photon beam energies above 10 MV. This interaction is not usually considered for patient treatments and is not discussed further in this chapter. More detail is given in Chapter 3.

2.4.5 The relative importance of the three main interactions

When photons interact with matter, there are three possible interactions, as discussed earlier. Which of these occurs depends on two things:

- The energy of the incident photon
- The atomic number (Z) of the material being interacted with

The probability of each interaction is denoted by a Greek letter:

τ for the photoelectric effect

σ for the Compton effect

K for pair production

Figure 2.6 shows the relative importance related to the atomic number of the absorber and the energy of the oncoming photons.

2.5 Attenuation: the exponential attenuation and the attenuation coefficient

As a beam of photons enters a material, it is attenuated.

The intensity emerging from the other side of the material is less than that entering the material.

The loss of intensity is proportional to the degree of intensity entering the material and proportional to the thickness of the material.

This can be written as:

$$\Delta I \propto -\Delta x . I_0$$

I_0 is the intensity of the photon beam at the point of entering the material. ΔI is a small change in intensity after passing through a small thickness, Δx of material. As

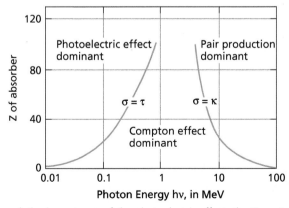

Figure 2.6 The relative importance of the photoelectric effect, the Compton effect, and pair production related to the Z of the absorber and the incident photon energy.

with all equations where two components are proportional to each other, a constant can be applied:

$$\Delta I = -\mu.\Delta x.I_0$$

μ is the total linear attenuation coefficient of the material and has the unit cm^{-1} or m^{-1}. It is the fractional reduction in intensity of a photon beam per unit length of the material. The equation assumes x is very small so for greater thickness the expression is integrated:

$$I_x = I_0 \exp(-\mu x)$$

where I_x is the intensity transmitted after the beam has passed through the material of x thickness.

We can derive the mass attenuation coefficient by dividing μ by the density of the material, ρ. The mass attenuation coefficient, μ/ρ, has units of m^2/kg or cm^2/gm. This gives the attenuation per unit mass rather than per unit path length. The relative importance of the three main interaction processes may be demonstrated by plotting the mass attenuation coefficient against photon energy (Figure 2.7).

2.5.1 Polyenergetic beams and broad beam geometry

The equation above holds true for a thin beam consisting of photons of a single energy. In 'real life', photon beams have a range of energies; the value of μ changes with the energy because the lower energy photons are preferentially absorbed earlier in the beam's journey through the material. Furthermore, the beams are broad, meaning there is greater scatter of photons as the beam passes deeper though the material. This has the effect of reducing the intensity *less* than expected, in other words there is less attenuation and more of the beam energy gets through than expected.

2.5.2 The half value layer

The half value layer (HVL) is the thickness of a material required to reduce the intensity of a beam by half.

Taking the equation defined above:

$$I_x = I_0 \exp(-\mu x)$$

If the initial intensity, I_0, is to be reduced by half =

$$I_0/2 = I_0 \exp(-\mu x)$$

x is the thickness of the material needed to reduce the intensity by half, that is the half value layer (HVL):

$$I_0/2 = I_0 \exp(-\mu \text{HVL})$$

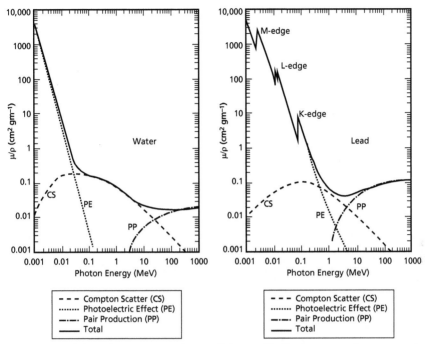

Figure 2.7 Variation of mass attenuation coefficients with photon energy for water and lead. Note the K, L, and M edges for lead corresponding to photo-electric absorption in the K, L, and M shells respectively.

Rearranging the equation gives:

$$HVL = \ln 2/\mu$$

that is,

$$HVL = 0.6931/\mu$$

The HVL is used to compare how penetrating the photon beams are. The more penetrating the beam, the greater the HVL. A penetrating beam is said to be 'hard'; it also serves as a description of the quality of the beam. Higher quality beams are harder and have larger HVLs, which really relate to the overall energy of the beam.

The concept of the half value layer can be applied to any factor, for example the tenth value layer being the thickness of material required to reduce the intensity of a beam to one-tenth of its original value and is often used in radiation protection calculations.

2.5.3 Mass energy transfer and mass energy absorption coefficients

We have explained the linear attenuation coefficient (μ) and mass attenuation coefficient (μ/ρ). They are particular to whatever material is attenuating a photon beam and have been defined for a wide range of materials, for example, water, bone, lead, etc. These coefficients also vary with energy, given that at different energy levels, different processes of photon–electron interaction occur (Figure 2.7). They relate to the reduction in *intensity* of a beam of photons.

The mass energy transfer coefficient describes the energy transferred from the beam to give kinetic energy to electrons in the medium. The mass energy absorption coefficient relates to how that kinetic energy is deposited in the medium.

This concept is revisited in Chapter 5, where 'mass energy transfer' is used for the calculation of kinetic energy released per unit mass (kerma) and 'mass energy absorption' is used in the calculation of radiation absorbed dose.

2.6 Photon offspring: the secondary electrons and their interactions

The photon interactions discussed earlier produce electrons (pair production) or impart energy to them. The electrons will, in turn, lose this energy in processes exactly equivalent to the electron interactions that occur in X-ray production:

♦ Excitation

♦ Ionization of an outer orbital electron

♦ Ionization of an inner orbital electron

♦ Production of bremsstrahlung

These interactions can be thought of as either collisions (ionization of orbital electrons) or radiative interactions (excitation and bremsstrahlung).

An electron, either given energy from a photon or created through pair production, will follow a path though the material. It will lose energy along the way through the four processes, until it stops. The point at which the electron stops varies according to the material through which it is travelling, and according to the energy the electron carries. Four features of this path can be defined (see Figure 2.8):

2.6.1 The path length

This is the absolute distance travelled by the electron as it passes through the material.

2.6.2 The range

This is the distance in the material over which energy is deposited. The range is effectively the depth of maximum penetration of a charged particle beam. For example, the path length and the range are very similar for all protons in a mono-energetic beam as they do not undergo wide angle scattering; they exhibit a pronounced Bragg peak (see section 3.3.1). However, electrons in a mono-energetic beam undergo lots of wide-angle scattering. While the electrons' path lengths might be similar, the range of the beam is more likely to be different and is dependent on the material and the energy the electron carries.

2.6.3 **The stopping power**

The '**stopping power**' describes a material's ability to stop an electron (or indeed any charged particle) and is the rate at which the electron loses its energy along its track. It relates to both the collision-type and the radiative-type interactions.

The unit of stopping power is Joules per metre (J m^{-1}).

The stopping power divided by the density of the material, gives the stopping power per unit mass of the material (J m^2 kg^{-1}).

2.6.4 **The linear energy transfer (LET)**

The linear energy transfer is the rate at which energy is deposited along a particle track. It is particle dependent and is different to stopping power. LET defines the amount of energy deposited in the material surrounding the particle track as opposed

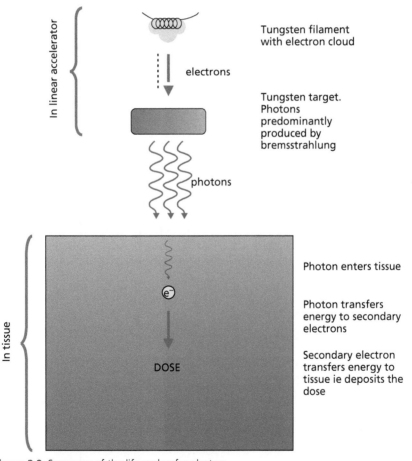

Figure 2.8 Summary of the life cycle of a photon.

to the amount of energy lost by the particle. Linear energy transfer therefore relates to the collision type interactions only. LET is usually expressed in units of keV per micrometre (keV μm⁻¹)

2.7 **The inverse square law**

A simple but important relationship, found in several areas of radiotherapy physics, is the inverse square law.

It states that that the dose rate (or dose) from a radiation source is proportional to the inverse of the square of the distance from the source. If the dose rate is *DR* and the distance is *d*, then:

$$DR \propto \frac{1}{d^2}$$

Looking at Figure 2.9, if we consider the intensity of radiation passing through an area A at a distance d from the source, as we move away from the source, the beam diverges. By the basic concept of similar triangles, as we move to a distance 2d, the area of the beam is now 4A. At a distance of 3d, the area of the beam is 9A. It can be thought of that the number of photons crossing the beam area A at distance d has to spread out to cover more area, so that the intensity at any point and hence dose rate or dose are similarly reduced. So as we move away from the source, the intensity of the beam at distance decreases by the square of the distance. Similarly, if we move closer

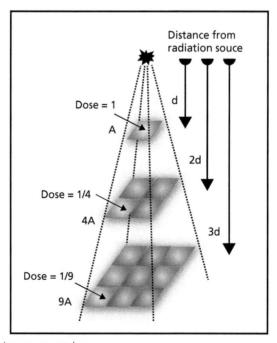

Figure 2.9 The inverse square law.

to the source, the dose rate or dose will increase. This can be demonstrated by shining a torch at a wall; as one moves the torch further away, the size of the light beam on the wall becomes both larger and fainter.

This rule works well if the source and point of measurement are both in air, but if there is any denser material present that will attenuate the beam, which needs to be accounted for separately.

It is usually applied in cases where the dose rate at one point is known and we want to know that dose rate at another. For example, if the dose rate at distance of 10 cm from a radiation source is 2 Gray per minute (Gy/min), if we move to a distance of 20 cm, what will the dose rate be?

$$\frac{DR_2}{DR_1} = \frac{d_1^2}{d_2^2}$$

If $DR_1 = 2$ Gy/min, $d_1 = 10$ cm and $d_2 = 20$ cm, then $DR_2 = 0.5$ Gy/min.

2.7.1 Focus-to-Surface Distance (FSD) or Source-to-Surface Distance (SSD)?

Note that the distance from the radiation source origin to the surface of the patient is usually referred to as the focus-to-surface distance (FSD). This is usually used when the radiation is produced by accelerating electrons, stopping them in a target, and the radiation arises from what is known as the focal spot. If the radiation originates from a radioactive isotope (or source) for example in a Cobalt machine (see section 11.5), then the term source-to-surface distance (SSD) is used. In practice, the terms FSD and SSD are the same thing, this being the distance from the origin of the radiation to the surface of the patient.

Chapter 3

Particles: Electrons, protons, and neutrons

Andrew Morgan and Andrew Nisbet

3.1 Introduction

The vast majority of radiotherapy treatments are performed using megavoltage photons, the physics of which have been discussed elsewhere in this book. For megavoltage photons the dominant interaction, Compton scattering, is with outer shell electrons of the atoms of the tissue, transferring energy to them, and it is these electrons which then move through tissue causing most of the damage to biological tissues. In particle therapy, be they electrons, protons, neutrons, or carbon ions, it is the *particles themselves* that either damage the tissue molecules directly or impart energy to electrons in the tissue.

Electron beams have been used in radiotherapy for many years. They can be used to treat superficial tumours without potentially damaging normal tissues lying at deeper depths. This is due to their rapid drop off in depth dose beyond the depth of maximum dose.

There is now considerable interest in the use of proton beams and carbon ion beams in the treatment of cancer. Their unique depth dose characteristics potentially result in the irradiation of less normal tissue than the most conformal photon treatments.

Fast neutron beams, using high energy neutrons, have been used in the past but fell out of favour due to unacceptable and unanticipated side effects. However, they can be present in high energy photon beams and the interactions they undergo are worthy of consideration. Boron neutron capture therapy, employing thermal neutrons, has also been the subject of a number of clinical studies.

Electrons, protons, and carbon ions are all charged particles. Neutrons are uncharged particles but can interact with nuclei in a material to produce potentially damaging charged particles so they are of relevance in this chapter. A proton may be considered a hydrogen nucleus with its electron removed. All 6 electrons must be removed from a carbon atom to produce a carbon ion.

Charged particles have an electric field associated with them and it is because of this field that charged particles lose energy when they travel through a medium. This lost energy is absorbed in the medium and can damage cellular DNA, leading to cell death—and so we have a potential means of treating tumours … but we're getting ahead of ourselves. We need to look at the interaction processes in a little more detail.

Uncharged particles, that is X-rays, gamma rays, and neutrons, lose energy in a different manner from that of charged radiations. Photons and neutrons may pass through matter with no interactions and therefore no energy loss. When they do lose energy, they tend to lose it in one or more discrete events such as a series of Compton-type interactions or a photo-electric absorption.

Charged particles, however, possess an electric field and they interact with the electrons or with the nucleus of virtually every atom which they pass. Such interactions are often referred to as Coulomb interactions, after a French physicist, Charles-Augustin de Coulomb, who first described the forces between charged particles in the 1780s. The probability of an uncharged particle passing through a layer of matter without interaction may be small but is finite. The probability of a charged particle passing through a layer of matter without interaction is zero. A single 10 MeV electron may undergo of the order of a million separate interactions before losing all of its kinetic energy.

The most important type of interactions which occur between a charged particle and an atom are illustrated below using a simple model. In this model, the atomic electrons exist in stable states of energy characterized by discrete levels surrounding the nucleus of an atom as discussed in Chapter 1.

3.2 Types of charged particle interactions

Charged particles can lose energy by three main processes when they pass through a medium. The mode of interaction is determined largely by the energy of the incident charged particle and by its distance of approach to the atom or nucleus (see Figure 3.1(a)). Consider the radius of the atom to be 'a'. The distance of closest approach to the nucleus is 'b', also known as the impact parameter. Note that in these examples, an electron is shown as the incident charged particle. E is the energy of the incident particle and ΔE is the energy lost to an atomic electron.

3.2.1 Soft collisions (where 'b' is greater than 'a')

If an electron passes an atom at a distance which is large compared to the size of the atom (Figure 3.1b), there are two possible interaction mechanisms:

1) Excitation of atomic electron to a higher level which returns to the ground state with emission of a photon.

2) Ionization of atom by excitation of valence shell electron. The net effect is the transfer of a few eV of energy to the medium.

It can be appreciated that large values of 'b' are more probable than 'hits' on individual atoms and therefore soft collisions are the most numerous type of charged particle interaction.

The absolute velocity of light in a vacuum is 3×10^8 metres per second. However, the velocity of light in a material such as water is less. While it is not possible to travel faster than the speed of light in a vacuum, it is possible for a highly energetic charged particle to travel at a velocity greater than the reduced speed of light in certain media. If such a medium is transparent then a very small part of the energy spent in soft collisions

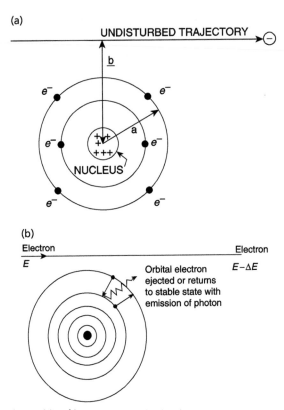

Figure 3.1 a. Relationship of impact parameter to atom.
Adapted with permission from Attrix, F. H. (2004) 'Introduction to Radiological Physics and Radiation Dosimetry' Fig. 8.1, p. 161. London: Wiley, VCH
b. Simple representation of soft collision.
Adapted from Klevenhagen, S C (1985) 'Physics of Electron Beam Therapy', Fig 2.1a, p. 38. Bristol: Adam Hilger

is emitted in the absorbing medium as a coherent bluish-white called Cerenkov radiation. The quantity of energy lost by Cerenkov radiation is less than 0.1% that lost by 'soft' collisions.

Cerenkov radiation has been cited as a reason for visual disturbances occasionally reported by patients undergoing radiotherapy close to the eye (Figure 3.2). High energy electrons may pass through the vitreous humour, resulting in Cerenkov production.

3.2.2 Hard collisions ('b' is roughly equal to 'a')

When 'b' is approximately equal to 'a', it is more probable that the incident electron will interact with one of the orbiting atomic electrons which is then ejected from the atom with significant kinetic energy (Figure 3.3a). This process is known as a hard collision. The ejected atomic electron is known as a delta ray (or δ-ray). Even though

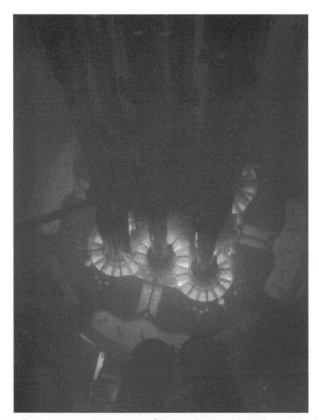

Figure 3.2 Nuclear reactor rods in a water filled cooling pond producing Cerenkov radiation.
Reproduced with permission from Argonne National Laboratory, Illinois

hard collisions are few compared to soft collisions, the fraction of energy lost by hard collisions is large and, overall, is roughly the same as that lost by soft collisions.

If an inner shell atomic electron is ejected, characteristic X-rays or Auger electrons are emitted which can result in energy being deposited away from the primary particle path.

An Auger electron can be considered to be the result of a characteristic X-ray being captured by an orbital electron and being ejected from the atom.

3.2.3 Radiative interactions with the nuclear electric field

If 'b' is (very) much less than 'a', an interaction takes place mainly with the nucleus and this is most important when the incident particle is an electron (Figure 3.3b). In about 95% of cases, the interaction with the nucleus is elastic. The electron's path will be changed, and it may lose a small but negligible amount of energy. Elastic nuclear interactions give rise to changes in the direction of the impinging electron but not to significant energy losses, so this is not a mechanism for transfer of energy to

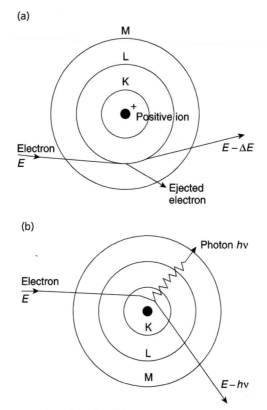

Figure 3.3 a. Representation of hard collision.
Adapted with permission from Klevenhagen, S C (1985) 'Physics of Electron Beam Therapy', Fig 2.1b, p. 38. Bristol: Adam Hilger.
b. Radiative interaction with a nuclear field.
Adapted with permission from Klevenhagen, S C (1985) 'Physics of Electron Beam Therapy', Fig 2.1c, p. 38. Bristol: Adam Hilger.

absorbing medium. It is an important means of scattering electrons and is the main reason why electrons follow tortuous paths, particularly in materials with a high atomic number, Z.

In the remaining cases, an inelastic interaction occurs. An electron passing near a nucleus may be deflected from its path by the action of the nuclear Coulomb force and lose energy. As the charged particle passes the vicinity of the nucleus, it suffers deflection and deceleration. As a result, part of its kinetic energy is dissociated from it and appears as a photon with energy hv (see section 1.4.5). The charged particle may give up to 100% of its kinetic energy as the photon. This process is known as *bremsstrahlung*—which is 'braking radiation' in German. The emitted radiation covers the entire spectrum of energies up to the maximum kinetic energy of the charged particle. The likelihood of a radiative interaction taking place depends on the square of the atomic number of the irradiated material (Z^2). It also depends inversely on the mass squared of the particle and so is considered insignificant for all charged particles, except electrons.

It should be noted that all photon beams, other than those from radio-isotopes, used in radiotherapy are generated by accelerating electrons to a high velocity and then stopping them suddenly to harvest the bremsstrahlung photons (see Chapter 2).

3.3 **Stopping power**

The rate at which a charged particle loses energy as it passes through a medium is known as the **stopping power**. The units of stopping power are given as Joules per metre as is usually shown by the term dE/dX—the rate of energy loss with distance travelled. Stopping power has collisional (due to soft and hard collisions) and radiative (due to Bremsstrahlung) components. For electron energies encountered in radiotherapy, radiative losses amount to about 1% of collisional losses in soft tissues. Bremsstrahlung-type interactions *may* occur in tissue but are not a significant source of dose to a patient.

dE/dX is called the linear stopping power. The term 'mass stopping power', often used in radiation dosimetry, refers to the linear stopping power divided by the density of the material through which the beam is passing.

3.3.1 **Variation of dE/dX with X**

A typical graph of dE/dX against distance travelled, X, for a single charged particle will look like that in Figure 3.4.

This type of graph is representative of the pattern of energy loss of every type of charged particle—not just protons! It is characterized by a relatively low and constant rate of energy loss immediately after entering a medium. However, towards the end of its path, the rate of energy loss rises dramatically and then falls to zero. This peak in the curve is known as the Bragg peak, after its discovery by William Henry Bragg in 1903.

The mathematical equation which describes the shape of the below curve is rather complex but there are a few important points which can be clearly stated.

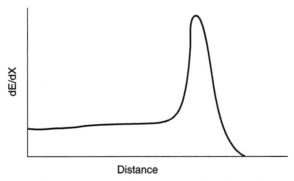

Figure 3.4 Variation of energy loss with distance for a charged particle.

The rate of energy loss with distance (dE/dX) is:

♦ Directly proportional to the square of the charge on the particle ... so an alpha particle which has a charge of + 2 will lose energy 4 times as fast as a proton which has a charge of + 1.

♦ Inversely proportional to the square of velocity of the charged particle ... as the particle slows down, the rate of energy loss increases—which fits in with the shape of the graph above.

♦ Independent of the mass of the charged particle—this means that for particles of the same energy, the rate of energy loss of a proton is the same as that of an electron as both have a charge of 1 unit.

Figure 3.5 shows the pattern of absorbed dose with depth from an electron beam and a proton beam. The characteristics appear to be completely different, but the energy loss of each particle type is exactly the same as shown in Figure 3.4. The reason relates to the relative mass of each particle. Electrons will undergo interactions with other electrons—which are the same mass—and will be easily scattered by the interactions undergone. Many will end up travelling in the direction they have come from—hence there is no well-defined Bragg peak for the beam as a whole. Protons on the other hand, having a mass nearly 2000 times greater than an electron are not easily deflected and an obvious Bragg peak is seen. Consider an electron as a ping-pong ball and imagine firing a ping-pong ball into a collection of other ping-pong balls—the

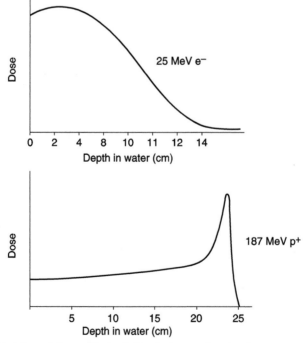

Figure 3.5 Variation of dose with depth for electron and proton beams.

original is unlikely to travel through the collection without deflection from its path. If you consider a proton as a ten-pin bowling ball and fire that at the same collection of ping-pong balls, it is easy to imagine that it would plough through them with minimal path deflection.

3.3.2 Restricted stopping power—where physics meets biology

This section describes the interface between the physics of radiotherapy and radio-biology, dealing with the deposition of energy on a microscopic level.

We have shown that charged particles generally lose energy in a large number of small interactions, each with small energy losses to atomic electrons via soft collisions. This is described as a 'continuous slowing down approximation' (CSDA). The energy lost by the charged particle in this way could be assumed to be transferred to the medium and be absorbed locally, that is within a small distance of its track through the medium, close, say, to a target of interest such as a DNA base pair. However, the situation is complicated by interactions that involve radiative losses and those that involve the production of delta rays.

Radiative losses produce photons which will deposit energy a long way from the point of interaction. Delta rays are energetic electrons (and so not really rays) resulting from large energy transfers to an atomic electron via hard collisions. The atomic electron is able to travel a distance and produce ionization far from its point of origin.

Therefore, the energy deposited by a charged particle in a given volume may be overestimated unless δ-ray equilibrium exists; that is for every δ-ray that leaves a small volume of material, a δ-ray enters the volume to replace the energy lost. This is not usually the case. Energy lost by a charged particle cannot necessarily be considered to be equal to energy deposited locally. Radiative losses and delta rays may be accounted for by using what is known as the **restricted collisional stopping power** which is usually simply called restricted stopping power to determine energy deposited locally. Radiative losses are ignored and only collisional losses, including some delta rays, that transfer up to a certain amount of energy which will be deposited close to the point of interaction are included in calculations. (See Figure 3.6).

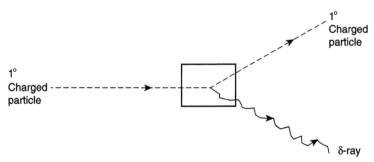

Figure 3.6 Energy loss from a small volume due to production of a delta ray.

Radiobiologists call restricted stopping power **linear energy transfer** (LET). LET represents the stopping power for all collisional interactions, including the production of δ-rays, up to a specified cut-off value. Interactions from radiative interactions are ignored as it is assumed that photons produced will interact with another electron a long way from the radiative interaction site.

It is important to appreciate that stopping power represents energy lost by a charged particle whereas LET represents energy absorbed locally.

Ionizing radiation interacts with matter in a similar way but different types of radiation differ in their effectiveness in damaging a biological system. The most important factor that influences the relative biological effectiveness of a type of radiation is the distribution of the ionizations and excitations in its path. The term linear energy transfer is used to describe both excitation and ionization events. The LET gives the average energy loss of a particle per unit length of travel in terms of keV/micrometre or keV/μm.

Given the shape of the curve shown in Figure 3.4, it can be appreciated that the LET of a particle will change with distance travelled. Commonly, LET values quoted are an average of energy lost with distance. The LET gives the average energy loss of a particle per unit length of travel. The variation of energy loss along the track of a charged particle has led to the utility of LET being questioned. However, the fact remains that it is a valuable method of comparing the energy deposition characteristics of different radiation modalities.

LET values vary from publication to publication, but the following may be taken as representative. All values quoted are in terms of keV/μm . An electron beam with a kinetic energy of 10 keV will have an LET of 2.5, whereas an electron beam with an energy of 1 MeV will have an LET of 0.2. Remember, the greater the energy, the greater the distance travelled, so the average for a given particle type will decrease with increasing kinetic energy. Proton beams of energy 10 MeV have an LET of around 5 while those of 100MeV have a value of around 0.5.

Alpha particles are relatively large and slow moving, so they will lose energy more quickly both because of the velocity and charge dependence on dE/dX. A 5.3 MeV alpha particle, such as emitted by polonium-210 has an LET of almost 50.

Neutrons are not directly ionizing themselves but they may cause a nucleus to break up, leading to the production of heavy charged nuclear fragments, with a correspondingly high LET.

The high LET exhibited by alpha particles is the main reason why the absorption of alpha-emitting isotopes into the human body is of great concern. They cause a great deal of damage to normal tissues and have been linked with the development of bone tumours.

Radium behaves in a similar way to calcium when ingested and is readily absorbed by bone where it may sit, irradiating bone marrow and other tissues. In 1917 the US Radium Corporation started producing a radium-containing paint called Undark, which, as the name may suggest, glowed in the dark. The company employed several thousand employees, mainly women, to paint Undark onto the hands and dials of watches. The employees were encouraged to keep the lines and characters they painted sharply defined by licking the tips of their brushes, thus continually ingesting small amounts of radium on a regular basis. Large numbers of the workers developed serious health issues including anaemia and mandibular necrosis resulting in tooth loss. Significant numbers went on to develop tumours.

3.4 **Neutrons**

Neutrons are not charged and hence are not directly ionizing but they interact quite readily with nuclei and can set protons and other nuclear fragments in motion by knock-on collisions. Photon interactions with matter almost always result in the production of high energy electrons, but neutron interactions with matter are highly complex and not readily categorized. There are several outcomes of neutron interactions but generally two processes are likely:

1) Elastic scattering

   A neutron interacts with a nucleus as whole. The nucleus gains kinetic energy and recoils through the medium. The original neutron loses energy and is deflected from its original path. The transfer of energy is greatest when the target nucleus is lightest, that is for hydrogen atoms.

2) Inelastic scattering

   Inelastic scattering is considered to occur when a neutron is absorbed by a nucleus, rather than scattering off it. This is where things start getting a little complex. The nucleus will then be unstable, and several different phenomena may occur to return it to a more stable state. It may eject one or more neutrons, which can then go on and interact with other nuclei. It may eject a proton, alpha particle, or larger nuclear fragment with high LET, depositing considerable energy and causing considerable normal tissue damage in the human body.

   The nucleus may also eject a high energy photon in order to return to a lower energy state.

   Following some unsuccessful clinical trials in the 1970s and 1980, neutron beams are no longer used, except for boron neutron capture therapy, where some interest remains. However, clinical photon beams may be contaminated with neutrons. How so?

3.4.1 **Neutron contamination of photon beams**

Clinical photon beams are produced by stopping high energy electron beams (see bremsstrahlung in section 2.3). The higher the energy of the electron beam, the higher the energy of the resulting photon beam. As discussed in Chapter 1, protons and neutrons are bound together in a nucleus and that binding energy is around 8 MeV per nucleon. If a photon with energy higher than 8 MeV is absorbed by a nucleus, a neutron can be ejected, in a process called a photo-nuclear interaction. This interaction mainly takes place with heavy nuclei, such as the heavy metals in the head of the treatment machine (tungsten and lead) at clinical photon energies above 10 megavolts (MV).

In practice, this issue is mostly limited to photon beams of 15 MV and greater, but neutrons can be detected in 10 MV beams. This can be a problem in the radiotherapy department for two reasons. First, the neutrons that escape the treatment machine create a radiation protection problem outside the room and secondly, the neutrons absorbed by the metals in the linear accelerator (linac) make those metals radioactive (see Chapter 1). Therefore, it is important for staff safety that treatment rooms containing high energy photon treatment units are adequately shielded against neutron leakage. The emission of a high energy photon following neutron absorption does not happen instantaneously. This 'induced radioactivity' may persist for several minutes after a high-energy photon treatment has finished, meaning that staff entering the treatment room may be exposed to a low intensity high energy photon field, posing a radiation protection issue.

The problem is more evident if a technical problem requires disassembly of the treatment head. The induced radioactivity in the vicinity of the linear accelerator target may mean that the commencement of service work may be delayed for several hours to allow dose rates to service personnel to reduce to acceptable levels.

3.5 Principles of heavier charged particle therapy

3.5.1 Protons

As discussed earlier, the rate of energy loss of all charged particles exhibits a characteristic shape, terminating in a Bragg peak.

Protons generally transfer energy to a medium in the same ways as electrons. They will undergo soft and hard interactions with atomic electrons as previously described and these represent the main source of energy loss. Radiative interactions are insignificant for protons and they will not undergo wide angle scattering like electrons but narrow angle scattering is possible due to Coulomb interactions with the nucleus. Protons, like neutrons, may also undergo inelastic collisions with nucleii, leading to the ejection of heavier nuclear fragments.

Protons are not easily deflected from their paths and so retain a distinctive Bragg peak at depth. The highly localized deposition of dose with minimal irradiation of normal tissues is a highly prized goal in radiotherapy and proton beams are of considerable use. However, for a mono-energetic proton beam, the Bragg peak can be so narrow that it is not clinically usable. While we aspire to miss normal tissues, missing the target is not an option.

There are two main ways by which this may be achieved and this depends on which method is used to produce the proton beams.

From Figure 3.7, the Bragg peak can be spread out into a plateau. The largest peak represents the highest energy of the beam. The lower peaks represent contributions from lower energy beams of different intensities, which when added together produce a plateau, meaning that tumours of appreciable thickness may be completely irradiated.

When it is not possible to vary the energy of the beam at the point of production, the energy of the beam incident on a patient may be varied by placing a rotating variable thickness wheel in the beam with open windows in it (Figure 3.8). When the

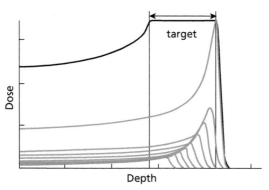

Figure 3.7 Spreading out a proton Bragg peak to cover a target.
Reproduced courtesy of Tony Lomax, Paul Scherrer Institute, Switzerland. Available at www.aapm.org/meetings/03SS/Presentations/Lomax.pdf

beam passes through the open part of the wheel, the protons incident on the patient are at maximum energy. When they pass through the thickest part of the wheel, they lose energy.

So, the beam which leaves the collimating system is a mixture of energies, the difference between the maximum and minimum energies being related to the thickness of the tumour to be treated. However, the beam modification is not yet complete. The rotating wheel will spread out the energy but do nothing to help shape the beam to conform to the tumour shape. The distal aspect of the tumour is usually closest to critical structures and we require a rapid dose fall off in this region. This is achieved by placing a compensator in the beam, which modulates its profile shape with depth to fit the shape of the target.

There is a major disadvantage to this method of production. While the dose can be conformed to the shape of the distal target volume, the spread of energies needed to cover the thickest part of the target cannot be changed laterally, meaning that if the

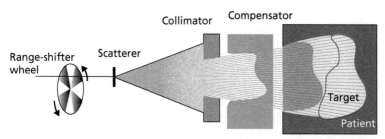

Figure 3.8 Use of a passive scatterer and compensator to conform dose to distal tumour limit.
Reproduced courtesy of Tony Lomax, Paul Scherrer Institute, Switzerland. Available at www.aapm.org/meetings/03SS/Presentations/Lomax.pdf

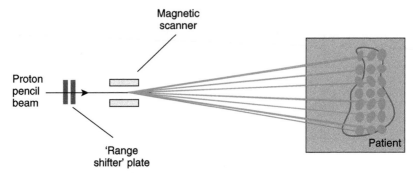

Figure 3.9 Representation of spot scanning for protons beams.
Reproduced courtesy of Tony Lomax, Paul Scherrer Institute, Switzerland. Available at www.aapm.org/meetings/03SS/Presentations/Lomax.pdf

tumour thickness changes laterally across the beam, there is generally an excess of normal tissue treated to a high dose on the proximal side of the target, as shown in Figure 3.8.

With newer technologies offering better beam energy control, it is possible to treat a large tumour by scanning a narrow proton beam though a tumour, changing the energy according to the depth required. This is known as spot scanning or active scattering. By moving the beam throughout the volume, a more conformal dose can be delivered to the proximal side of the target volume.

As with more conventional forms of photon radiotherapy, consideration needs to be given to patient and organ motion during treatment. Spot scanning (also known as intensity modulated proton therapy (IMPT)) offers the potential for more conformal doses but also presents the risk of missing the tumour due to organ or patient motion during treatment (Figure 3.9). The more 'barn door' approach of passively scattered broad beams reduces conformality, the risk of geographic miss of a moving target is reduced. However, recently the technique of gated therapy (see section 9.11.1) using spot proton beams has been developed and all new installations are now of the spot scanning type.

It has been demonstrated that beams produced by passive scattering have a higher neutron contamination than those generated by spot scanning and are hence considered less appropriate for the treatment of paediatric tumours.

3.5.2 Carbon ions

Carbon ions are also of potential interest in cancer treatment. Being about 12 times heavier than a proton, they suffer even less lateral scattering and have a narrower lateral penumbra than protons. However, the dose deposited by carbon ions does not fall off as quickly as protons after the Bragg peak. This is due to nuclear fragmentation, with lighter ions being produced in these nuclear reactions that have a larger penetration due to being lighter, hence creating a dose tail at the distal side of the Bragg peak.

Chapter 4

Putting the IT in RT

Niall MacDougall and Andrew Morgan

4.1 Introduction

In this chapter, we address the whole process of modern radiotherapy (RT) from introduction of patient demographic data into a Hospital Information System, through imaging associated with target definition, treatment planning and delivery, to end of treatment and eventually follow-up, as it works 'under the bonnet' in a fully electronic department. Also provide a simple set of references for all information technology (IT) concepts that occur in the book. If we can do this without losing you, then we'll be very happy!

We shall demystify frequently used terms such as DICOM, IP addressing, databases and The Cloud. From this point we should be able to demonstrate the possibilities and benefits of modern RT IT systems, but also the potential pitfalls and dangers that might befall the unwary.

4.2 Computers, who needs them?

Modern RT departments cannot function without IT support. Even up to the early 1990s, much of the data used in the RT treatment planning and delivery processes had to be manually entered into the relevant computer systems. Most data produced by RT treatment planning systems were printed and then manually typed into the linear accelerator. This was a time-consuming process, was prone to errors, and put a limit on the amount of data that could be used for a patient treatment. Things started to change in the mid-1990s with the introduction of multi-leaf collimators and the more widespread use of computed tomography (CT) images in treatment planning. However, rapid increases in computing power have helped to transform RT, allowing large amounts of data to be accessed and highly complex mathematical models to be run to efficiently calculate the radiation doses to be delivered (intensity modulated RT (IMRT), volumetric modulated arc therapy (VMAT), image-guided RT (IGRT)). The next computer developments are already with us, with the harnessing of Artificial Intelligence (AI) allowing online adaptive treatments and computer-assisted contouring.

4.2.1 Computers are everywhere

Imaging investigations—magnetic resonance imaging (MRI), CT, positron emissions tomography (PET), ultrasound, etc.—all generate images through the use of computers, indeed none of these imaging techniques would be possible if it were not for the calculating power of computers. Although generating an image is only the start, we now have the problem of how to get these images off the CT scanner in a way that they can be read by another computer. In former times, the CT images would be printed onto a sheet of film. The person looking at them could easily tell that 'Mr Patient' was the patient's name and 'R1400400' was the hospital number. They could then look at all the pictures of the CT slices printed below and gain all the information they needed from the CT scans. However, we don't have to emphasize the advantage of not having to generate and store all that printed film. Anyone that has worked (or had to access historical data) in a paper- and film-based department will know of the limitations.

So, we want to do all this electronically, which makes accessing data easier, but setting everything up is a little bit more complex.

Computers are not yet as smart as a person so cannot reliably tell a name from another piece of information, such as a hospital number. Also, printed pictures contain a lot of information, which is takes a lot of electronic space to store. So, we have to get a bit clever to make this all work efficiently.

4.3 Data communication

One of the oldest problems of mankind is that of communication. The ability to convey information concisely and accurately is one that is highly valued. Just as one person talking to another must speak the same language, so computers talking to each other must talk in a similar 'language'. However, the analogy can be stretched further, even if two people speak the same language, different regional dialects can impede communication resulting in misunderstanding!

Now, keep that image in mind as we stretch the imagination to make computing a simpler topic to understand.

Back in the dim and distant past (before DICOM—see below) all medical equipment talked in a local 'in-house' style. To use the human analogy, each had their own language. So, for example, if we put a 'Manufacturer X' MRI image onto a 'Manufacturer Y' reviewing station, nothing would be displayed unless one could write a translator program to make the file readable.

4.3.1 DICOM

DICOM (Digital Imaging and Communication in Medicine) is a structured way of communicating electronic information. The DICOM file is a standard form (like an application form for a passport) that the sending computer fills in before attaching the image to the end (Table 4.1). From the example in the previous paragraph if we introduce DICOM, Manufacturer X and Manufacturer Y both agree that their imaging systems will write and read data in the same way: according to the DICOM standard. Now there should be no need for translation: the sending computer orders the information in exactly the way the receiving computer expects to see it. As the receiving computer, I know the first thing I will see is the patient's surname, so I know that whatever is written there is that value.

But, simply put, a DICOM image file starts with a 'header' which is just text that contains all the relevant details pertaining to the patient, hospital, and imaging modality.

Table 4.1 Simplified example of a DICOM file

Property Name	Data
StudyDate	20110404
Modality	RTImage
PatientName	PatientA
PatientID	123456

ImageData

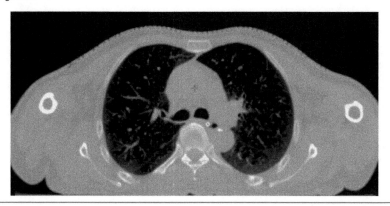

At the end of the text comes the image (e.g. the CT slice), which is compressed to save space in tagged image file format (TIFF). If you imagine this like a Word document with a patient report and a picture at the bottom, you'd be close!

If you're surprised, don't be. It really is this basic. And there is more than one type of DICOM, so it is not enough for a device to be 'DICOM compatible', it must be the 'right kind of DICOM' compatible. This is potentially a source of error that could affect patient treatment. So, we've packed up the images in a nice parcel, now to get them to the RT department.

All modern imaging techniques produce images that are in the DICOM format. All the image types that might go into an RT treatment planning system (such as CT, MRI, and PET) are in DICOM format. The headers for each image type will all be slightly different, but that doesn't matter. DICOM means that the planning system can understand the content of the headers and present the images to the user in the correct format.

There are 5 main sub-formats of DICOM for RT (Table 4.2 and Figure 4.1). To demonstrate their use, let's assume that we have a series of CT images on a planning system. Generally, the first thing that happens is that some outlines are drawn. These are usually the target volumes and critical organs. There are several mechanisms for performing contouring and the fine details are not important. What is important is that at the end of the process, we have a set of contours on which a plan can be designed. This set of contours can be stored in what is known as DICOM-RT (RT structure set)

Table 4.2 Radiotherapy DICOM objects

DICOM RT object	Main property	Example contents
RT Structure Set	Patient anatomical information	PTV, OAR, other contours
RT Plan	Instructions to the linac for patient treatment	Treatment beam details, e.g. gantry, collimator, and couch angles; jaw and MLC positions
RT Image	Radiotherapy image storage/ transfer	Planning CT, portal image, cone beam CT, etc.
RT Dose	Dose distribution data	Patient dose distributions (in 3D), dose volume histograms.
RT Treatment Record	Details of treatment delivered to patient	Date and time of treatment, MU delivered actual linac settings.

format. So the patient record now contains a set of DICOM images and a DICOM-RT structure set which contains details on the number of contours drawn, number of points in each contour, and their names. The next step is to put some beams on the plan.

This process generates another DICOM-RT file called the RT-Plan, which contains details of each treatment beam, such as its name, jaw settings, energy, monitor units, etc.

Once the beams have been positioned, a dose calculation is usually done and as you might well have already guessed, this generates a DICOM-RT file called RT-Dose. This contains details of the dose calculation matrix geometry, dose volume histogram data, etc.

At some point during the planning process, digitally reconstructed radiographs may be produced and there is a DICOM-RT format for these called RT-Image. Verification images taken using an electronic portal imaging device also generate images in RT-Image format.

When the plan is ready for treatment, some or all these files may be sent to the linear accelerator control system. The RT-Plan is essential in this respect but some of the others are optional and the functionality available may be vendor specific. Every time the patient has treatment, the treatment parameters used are stored by a **record and verify system.** Again, at the end of treatment, the full treatment record can be stored as our fifth type of RT DICOM object: an RT-Treatment Record (Table 4.2).

4.3.2 **Record and verify systems**

A record and verify system (R&V system) is a database with various bits of software which allow most of the functions in RT to occur. R&V systems are named from the days when all they were used for was to record delivered treatments and ensure the same treatment got delivered from one day to the next. The computer systems used today are much more sophisticated, allowing all kinds of information to be added to

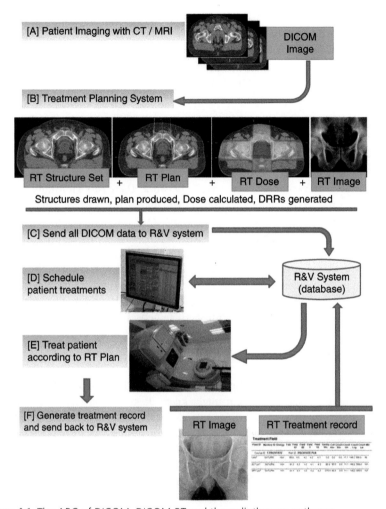

Figure 4.1 The ABC of DICOM. DICOM-RT and the radiotherapy pathway.

the patient record, such as diagnosis, treatment plans, imaging, etc. The list is almost endless.

So where is this obsession with DICOM going? The major advantage of the adoption of an international standard such as DICOM is to increase the longevity of all patient data stored electronically. All equipment manufacturers provide mechanisms for backing up and archiving data. However in the pre-DICOM years all such data were stored in a manufacturer specific format, meaning that it couldn't be interpreted by another manufacturers' equipment. This might not seem much of a problem but, for example, when a department changed its planning system, physicists were usually left to destroy a pile of tapes or other media containing data from the old system which couldn't be used on the new one! Now, if all manufacturers implement DICOM uniformly, this scenario will be unlikely to arise as the data from the old system will be readable by the new one (or by another manufacturer's system in different hospital). This means that if a patient undergoes treatment in one centre, then moves house and requires treatment later in another centre, the old record is accessible and transferrable to the treating centre so the previous RT can be safely accounted for in the new treatment.

4.4 Networking

A single computer sitting by itself is of some use but if a computer can communicate with other computers, its potential use increases manyfold. A group of computers that communicate with each other is known as a **network**. There isn't a minimum number of computers needed to define a network—there may be just 5 or 500 (the Internet is just a big network). The important matter is that they communicate with each other quickly and efficiently, getting data to where the information needs to be in a timely manner. In a hospital environment, computers are generally connected by a physical network—usually a cable. The methods of connecting computers with cables are too numerous to describe but one of the simplest ways is to connect computers using a device known as a **hub**. A hub is simply a box which cables from all computers go to and which enables computers to transfer data between each other (analogous to a crossroad).

4.4.1 IP addressing

In order to transfer data between computers, they need to know each other's identities. While the humans operating them might know them as 'The Planning System' or 'Linac 1 PC', the computers use a different notation known as an IP (Internet Protocol) address. This is usually a 12-digit number, made up of four groups of three numbers separated by full stops. A typical example might be 105.234.100.185. Each group of three numbers must be within the range 0–255. This gives a possible 4.3 billion IP addresses. On any given network, each computer must have a unique IP address or things get very confused. It's a bit like giving critical instructions to two people called Bob: 'So, Bob, I'd like you to carry out activity X and Bob, I'd like you to carry out activity Y. Clear? Good.' Neither Bob knows what they're meant to be doing and so will probably do nothing, or both try to do it and conflict with each other. It is the responsibility of the network manager to make sure that each system is allocated a unique IP address.

4.4.2 Data storage

A device that's generally also associated with a network is a **server**. It is possible for users to store data on each computer they use. However, there are very good reasons for not doing so:

1) If users then move to another computer, they may not be able to access the data they were working on previously

2) If the computer malfunctions or breaks down, data being worked on may be lost

3) If the computer gets stolen, data may be lost, and if the data identifies patient re-lated information, there will be mountains of paperwork to fill in and jobs may be lost!

Therefore it is common practice to use a data server. A server is a computer a bit like a bigger version of your desktop computer but with some extra parts and features to enable it to continue working if one individual part of it fails. It also runs software which allows many users to access it simultaneously. So a server gets around the above problems, because:

1) all users can access the server
2) the server creates several copies of the data stored on it so if one part fails, backup copies already exist
3) the server is located in a locked cabinet in a restricted access room so the chances of it being stolen are minimized.

There may well be more than 1 server on a network. Servers are designed to attempt to protect data integrity. Most PCs have 1 hard disc where data are stored. If that hard disc fails, all data stored on it are likely to be lost—or at least corrupted in some way. Servers use what is known as a RAID architecture—Redundant Array of Independent Discs. All data stored on them are copied and shared between several independent hard discs (minimum of 2 discs). The server controller knows where all the data are stored—if one disc fails, it can easily be replaced and the data that were stored on it is restored from other discs in the RAID. Of course, this is absolutely no use if someone steals the complete server, which is why such devices are usually stored in remote, secure rooms with restricted access. In some cases, additional security may be pro-vided when data are exceptionally important, by copying that data (mirroring) to an-other server in a different geographic location.

4.4.3 Simple network layout

Having introduced the main elements of a network, let's look at how a typical small network may be represented (Figure 4.2).

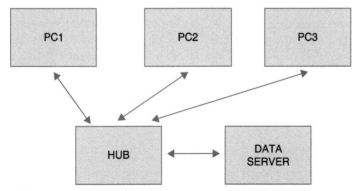

Figure 4.2 Generic representation of computer network.

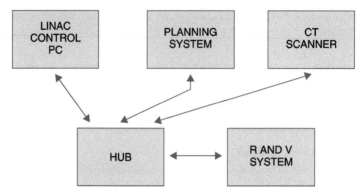

Figure 4.3 Generic representation of simple radiotherapy network.

In a typical RT department, this may equate to what is in Figure 4.3.

So, putting it simply, patients will have a planning CT scan. The CT scans will be sent to the treatment planning system where a plan will be produced. The treatment plan will be sent to the R&V system where it forms the basis for the patients' RT treatment record. From here, the necessary linear accelerator (linac) parameters and dose data are transferred to the treatment unit computer on a daily basis for treatment. Any treatment amendments or notes can be added to the record and stored back on the R&V system for recall the following day.

These diagrams represent very simple networks and in larger departments, such diagrams will get very complex once we've added in other equipment such as portal imaging devices, cone beam CT units, and other imaging devices such as CT, MRI, and PET scanners. However, the basic principles will remain the same as described earlier. Each computer system on the RT network needs to be assigned an IP address to enable it to communicate with other computers on the network.

4.4.4 The cloud

Let's now stretch the diagram of the network (in Figure 4.4) so that we move the 'R&V system' to a different building, possibly in a different city. Now, instead of the RT department owning the R&V system server, let's pay someone else (a company or individual) to use one of their servers. We can effectively rent server space from a company and run the RT department from there. This is 'the cloud': someone else's server. There are pros and cons to this approach which need to be carefully assessed. One pro is that access to cloud systems will reduce the need for complex hardware on site, meaning that expensive hardware upgrades may be avoided. Among the cons is the big issue of possible 'third party' control of patient data and guaranteed security of and access to that data.

4.4.5 Network security

One prospect that terrifies IT and RT Physics Departments alike is the potential for introducing computer viruses onto a network. Most computer systems use

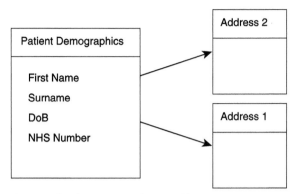

Figure 4.4 Simple example of a patient with two addresses.

Windows software and are potential targets for malicious software writers. Viruses can be quite easily and usually quite innocently introduced into a department. Staff often work at home on computers which may be infected and transfer the virus to a network via a memory stick or similar device. Once a file is opened on the network, it spreads to other computers. Most viruses can be easily dealt with by virus-checking software which warns users of any threat. However, some systems cannot run anti-virus software. For example, computers that are provided with linear accelerators and treatment planning system manufacturers are considered to be 'medical devices'. These were developed and tested by the suppliers without any anti-virus (AV) software present on them as AV software may cause the systems to malfunction: there are many different AV software packages and it is not possible to test them all. Therefore medical devices must be protected and this is often by use of a **firewall**. A firewall is a box (a bit like a hub) that sits on the network between the medical device computer and the rest of the network, like a bouncer on a nightclub door. It has rules about what it will and will not allow to pass through it, so in theory it will allow computers to do what is expected of them, but block the sorts of activities which viruses might initiate. Other methods of reducing the risk of virus introduction include disabling the use of CDs and USB ports for memory sticks and blocking access to the Internet. Many RT departments have experienced computer virus outbreaks and the impact can be devastating, occasionally stopping patient treatment for days.

4.5 **Patient safety**

Perhaps one of the greatest benefits of computing in RT is the reduction of transcription errors (by only storing information in one place). The RT pre-treatment process involves many different groups of staff adding new information and modifying existing information on the patient's treatment plan. If one is to carry this out manually, then an accurate patient treatment relies on all staff concerned transcribing important information with no errors from one piece of paper to another. This can be particularly troublesome with numbers and decimal places.

If one can generate the information for patient treatment on the planning system and then save it on a server that all other staff, and the linear accelerator, can access, then there is no need for anyone to copy any important data. But how do we store all this information electronically in a way that is safe and accurate? We use software called a **database**.

4.5.1 Databases

Don't give up at this point just because of the title! Databases are quite simple beasts, if we don't get too technical. The main aim here is to store information in an orderly manner (so you can find it again) with no repetition. The best way to keep an accurate record of a piece of information and be able to update it is if there is only one copy of it. At a basic level, a database is a way of storing large amounts of related data in the simplest way possible. There is lots of complex maths behind this, but let's not go there. If we consider the information required to treat a patient with RT, this should all be self-explanatory.

In a patient's paper notes (if you still have them!), every piece of paper should have a patient ID sticker on it. This will contain information unique to the patient: first name, surname, ID number, address. This is a sensible approach, for if an important piece of paper (e.g. prescription card) is dropped from the patient folder it will be instantly identifiable and easily reunited with the patient notes. However, what if we discover that the patient's ID number on the ID sticker is incorrect (due to a data-entry problem)? There may be tens (or hundreds) of stickers on the notes, treatment plan, images, etc., and we'll have to manually correct every one of them.

However, if this information is stored in a database, then it can contain all the information in the notes, but organized to store each unique piece of information in one place only. As such, in its storage form, it would not make much sense. However, the database is a bit cleverer.

If we consider the patient's ID sticker. We would store the information to generate unique patient IDs using the following identifiers:

♦ Unique identifiers (that cannot be changed), for example name, date of birth, National Health Service (NHS) number, and hospital number. We store this information together in a 'demographic table'.

♦ Identifiers that can be changed by the patient, for example telephone number and address. We store these in an 'address table'.

We then link these together, for example the demographic table can have many address tables.

We are saying that whilst a patient can only have one copy of the demographic table (therefore only one date of birth (DoB), name, etc.) they can have many copies of the Address table. Therefore, more than one address, phone number, etc. These two tables are joined together and the join knows this rule. This rule is a relation, which makes a *relational database* (albeit a very simple one). This concept can be easily expanded to include the course of treatment (patients can have many courses), each course can have many phases, etc.

By storing the patient's data in this way we only have to store (or change) information in one place. So, if we enter Marjory Bloggs' particulars into this database and you are about to authorize a completed electronic treatment plan, but, oops, you notice we've spelt her name wrong! You can change it in one place and all the multiple plans, images, etc. will now be linked to this new name you have entered. This is an improvement on changing 30 ID labels in the paper example. Press print and any paper reports will come out correct too.

The possibilities, from this simple start, are almost endless. At a press of a button you can retrospectively gather all kinds of information from clinical trial data to workload figures. However, it is important to stress that if you don't put the information in at the start, then it won't be there later.

The cynical reader may be thinking 'so very good, you have all the information in one place and once it is stored the patient's treatment will always be the same day after day. Well, what if it is stored incorrectly?'

This is a very real problem. Computers can ensure consistency, but it is the job of clinical staff to ensure what is stored there is correct from the start. To this end there are many checking procedures that occur in a patient's route to treatment in RT. This is the case if the treatment is paper-based or electronic.

4.6 **Summary**

Reading this chapter won't make you an IT expert but it should remove some of the fear of dealing with electronic issues in an RT department. The central message is that whilst IT has enabled RT to be immeasurably more sophisticated it is not always as turn-key as one would desire.

Chapter 5

Dosimetry: Measuring radiation dose

Tony Greener and John Byrne

5.1 Introduction

Accurate determination of dose is crucial. Errors in dose determination can cause failure of tumour control or unacceptable normal tissue damage. Accurate determination is vital in clinical trials where the assumption is made that the observed response has been caused by delivery of a particular dose. Dose measurement is difficult but for effective radiotherapy, it needs to be better than 5% accurate.

Radiation emanates from a source, travels a distance, and then interacts with the material through which it is travelling, resulting in deposition of dose. When a dose measurement is made, the value obtained from the device is an indication of the energy deposited in the device itself and not to the patient or material in which the device sits. It is important to understand how the output of the measuring device (detector) is converted to the dose that would have been delivered to that point in the medium in which the detector sits. This can be understood by learning the concepts of absorbed dose, exposure, and kerma, and the relationship between them, explained below.

5.1.1 Absorbed dose

Dosimetry defines a numerical relationship between ionizing radiation and the effect that it produces. This effect will vary according to the amount of energy deposited within a material of a given mass. Likewise, for the same amount of energy deposited, the effect would differ if the energy were deposited within a larger, or smaller, mass of material. The definition of absorbed dose is simply the expression of these observations.

The unit of absorbed dose is defined by the International Commission on Radiation Units (ICRU) (see section 9.8.1) as the energy absorbed (E) per unit mass (m).

$$D = E/m$$

In SI units this is Joules per kilogram ($J \ kg^{-1}$) and is given the special name Gray (Gy). When prescribing a dose of 50 Gy it could in principle also be prescribed in fundamental units as 50 $J \ kg^{-1}$. The Gray is small when compared with other more obvious examples of energy dissipation. For a tumour of mass 100 g (0.1 kg) a total dose of 50 Gy results in a deposited energy of only $50 \times 0.1 = 5$ Joules. This is comparable to that delivered to a 1 kW heater in only 5 milliseconds. The heating effect of ionizing radiation per Gy is very small with the temperature rises in irradiated tissues resulting from typical clinical doses being less than 0.001 ˚C (0.00024 ˚C per Gy for water). Calorimetry, the measurement of such temperature rises, although technically challenging is the only method of directly determining absorbed dose. This methodology is discussed later. There is a clear relationship between tumour control probability (TCP) and absorbed dose (see section 15.3.1) so it is best to quantify the delivery of radiotherapy by prescribing in terms of absorbed dose.

Accurate and traceable dose determination is crucial in maintaining consistency between different treatment equipment within a single department as well as maintaining consistency between equipment in different departments nationally and internationally. Clinical trials and the adoption of clinical protocols implicitly rely on the consistency of dose measurement.

5.1.2 **Exposure**

The way in which absorbed dose has been quantified has been governed by the radiation energies involved and the technology available to quantify them. The first radiation quantity to be defined was exposure. This concept relies on the number of ionization events measured as an indication of deposited energy in a medium. The greater the energy deposited, the greater the dose. The definition of exposure has undergone many refinements over the years, but the most recent definition is:

> The unit of exposure (X) is defined as the quotient Q/m where Q is the total charge of the ions (of one sign) produced in air when all electrons liberated by photons in air of mass m are completely stopped in air.

$$X = Q/m$$

In SI units this is Coulombs per kilogram (C kg^{-1}) where coulomb is the SI unit of charge.

The definition of exposure specifically mentions air as the material in which the ions are produced, that they are completely stopped and concerns only photon radiation. The effective atomic number (Z) of air (7.64) is similar to that of water and soft tissue (7.42). This is important when considering measurements in low kilovoltage (kV) energy ranges when the photoelectric effect is dominant (proportional to Z^3).

5.1.3 **Kerma: kinetic energy released per unit mass**

All dose is delivered by charged particles (electrons in this case). Photons need to kick electrons into action to deliver dose. This initial kick is called kerma.

Photons are not directly ionizing. They do not possess charge and only transfer energy to the irradiated material via Compton, photoelectric, or pair production processes. These interactions produce a charged particle, be it a recoil electron (Compton), liberated electron (photoelectric), or electron and positron pair (pair production). The charged particles then impart energy to the material through collisional losses. The concept of kerma was introduced to describe the first part of this two-stage process and is defined as:

$$K = E_{tr} / m$$

where E_{tr} is the sum of the initial kinetic energies of all the charged particles liberated by uncharged particles in a mass m. Kerma is an acronym for Kinetic Energy Released per unit Mass. The unit of kerma is Joules per kilogram ($J\,kg^{-1}$), which, as for absorbed dose, is given the special unit of Gray (Gy).

Kerma differs from exposure in that it can be defined for any material, not just air. A statement of kerma is not complete without defining the material concerned.

5.2 The relationships between exposure, kerma, and absorbed dose

5.2.1 Exposure and kerma

Air kerma quantifies the *transfer* of energy whereas exposure quantifies the *absorption* of energy required to liberate a certain amount of charge via ionization of air molecules. Exposure can be measured directly but kerma cannot. However, the relationship between exposure and air kerma is straightforward and indicates how air kerma can be derived from an exposure measurement.

$$K_{air} = X.(W/e)\ Gy$$

W/e is a constant, of value 33.97 $J\,C^{-1}$, and is the energy required to create a charge of 1 C in air.

Determination of air kerma is all very well but few patients are made from air! From a dosimetry perspective the ideal patient is one made entirely from water and so we are more interested in water kerma.

Before looking at the relationship between kerma and absorbed dose we need to introduce 2 more quantities. A source of ionizing radiation gives rise to a radiation field; particle fluence and energy fluence are 2 quantities used to characterize the radiation field. Within the radiation field there will be a flow or fluence of particles (Φ), defined as the number of particles (N) incident on a sphere of cross-sectional area (a). Fluence is defined as:

$$\Phi = N/a \quad SI\,units\ m^{-2}$$

A sphere is chosen rather than a plane area so that the presented cross-sectional area is the same from all directions. Particle fluence is therefore independent of radiation direction.

Instead of just the number of particles we could consider the energy carried by these particles. The energy fluence (Ψ) is defined as the radiation energy (R) entering a sphere of cross-sectional area (a):

$$\Psi = R/a \quad SI\,units\,J\,m^{-2}$$

5.2.2 **Kerma and absorbed dose**

Remember that absorbed dose is the energy absorbed per unit mass to a medium whereas kerma is the energy transferred from photons to charged particles within that medium. Considering a thin layer of material, represented by the dotted lines in Figure 5.1, we can demonstrate the problem that needs to be resolved to equate kerma and absorbed dose. In this explanation we will only consider photons as the incoming radiation, and electrons as the charged particles. Incoming photons may interact at any point within the medium. The kinetic energy released at the interaction point is represented by E_{tr}. We can see that, for an interaction in the layer between the dashed lines, some of the energy transferred will be expended through collisional losses and absorbed within this layer but some, represented by E_{out}, will be imparted beyond this layer. The amount of energy E_{out} does not contribute to the absorbed dose within the dashed layer. For a single photon interaction this represents a problem as kerma and absorbed dose will never be the same in this region. However, in a realistic situation there will be many similar photon interactions occurring throughout the irradiated volume.

Some interactions occurring outside the region of interest result in energy being deposited within the layer (E_{in}). On average the kinetic energy lost (E_{out}) from electrons leaving the thin layer will be balanced by the kinetic energy gained from electrons entering the thin layer i.e. $E_{out} = E_{in}$. The absorbed dose or net kinetic energy imparted to this layer can be written as:

$$\text{Dose} = \text{Total energy transferred} - E_{out} + E_{in}$$

If we assume that the condition described above holds and that the total energy in and out are the same, we arrive at:

$$\text{Dose} = \text{Total energy transferred}$$

By equating the charged particle energy entering to that energy leaving we have assumed that a situation called **charged particle equilibrium** (CPE) exists in the region

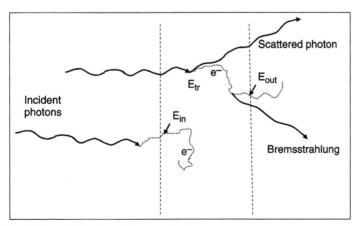

Figure 5.1 Relationship between kerma and dose.

of interest. So, on the assumption that CPE exists we arrive at the conclusion that the absorbed dose in a medium (D_{med}) is equal to that energy transferred and absorbed locally through collisions (K_{coll}).

$$D_{med} = K_{coll} \quad \text{assuming CPE}$$

Under conditions of CPE absorbed dose is equal to collision kerma. For X-ray energies below about 300 keV the radiative losses due to bremsstrahlung are negligible (i.e. Krad ≈ 0) so that absorbed dose and kerma are taken as the same. However, the relationship between kerma and dose becomes more complex as the photon energy increases to the megavoltage (MV) range. The concept of CPE as expressed here is somewhat simplified and is difficult to achieve in MV beams. The closest we get to CPE is at the point of dose maximum. Beyond this, the kerma and dose curves separate by a distance that depends on the beam energy and a condition known as transient charged particle equilibrium (TCPE) exists. TCPE can be used instead of CPE with suitable correction factors. The relationship between kerma and dose is discussed further in section 6.3.

5.2.3 Electronic equilibrium

The special condition of CPE (also called electronic equilibrium) is an important concept in radiation dosimetry. Electronic equilibrium exists if the number of electrons entering a space is the same as the number exiting and if their energies are similar. Why is electronic equilibrium so important and what are the consequences when it does not occur?

As stated earlier, a primary goal in dosimetry is to determine the dose at a point in the medium as it would be if the detector used to perform the measurement wasn't there. The method of correcting for this assumes the presence of the detector does not disturb CPE in the medium (see section 5.8.2).

Disruption in CPE is most frequently caused by a step change in the material the photons are interacting with. This is an issue for clinical treatment plans as well as for dosimeters. A good example of this is radiation passing through muscle into bone (Figure 5.2).

Consider the regions immediately each side of the interface between the two different materials in Figure 5.2. They are close enough to each other that we can assume that the number of photons per unit area is the same. The kerma on each side of the interface will differ depending on how readily photons interact with each material; the more interactions that occur, the more electrons are set in motion and the higher the kerma. This depends on things such as the photon energy as well as atomic number and electron density of the materials considered. This change in kerma is in proportion to the mass energy transfer coefficients (see section 2.5.3) of the two materials and therefore produces a step change in kerma at the boundary. As the kerma changes, so does the absorbed dose on each side of the boundary, this time according to the ratio of the mass energy absorption coefficients of the two materials. Note that while the kerma curve changes in a discrete step, the dose changes

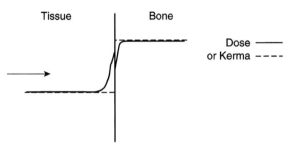

Figure 5.2 Dose and kerma at a tissue interface.

more gradually. The increase in dose in muscle close to the bone is due to electrons being back-scattered from the higher density bone to the right. The increase in dose in bone is due to the build-up effect, similar to when a photon beam passes from air to soft tissue, and is described in Chapter 6. Such interfaces provide examples of electronic disequilibrium. Interfaces are clinically important in treatment planning but are the hardest to model accurately.

These build-up/build-down dose modelling changes close to interfaces provide a challenge for computer planning algorithms to model dose in these regions. This can lead to inaccuracies in these regions, if not using up-to-date algorithms. This issue can become more pronounced at higher energies. Practical examples of this include secondary build up in the superficial layers of the larynx between the air and larynx wall. A similar effect can also occur for lung patients, particularly if a large volume of low-density lung is traversed immediately before the tumour. This particular example is discussed further in Chapter 9. To reduce these effects a lower beam energy (e.g. 6 MV) would be chosen.

5.3 Absorbed dose in different tissues and materials

5.3.1 Mass energy absorption coefficients

The energy absorbed per unit mass in two different materials, subjected to the same photon fluence, will be in proportion to their mass energy absorption coefficients. The ratio of mass energy absorption coefficients is:

$$(\mu_{en}/\rho)_{med}/(\mu_{en}/\rho)_{air}$$

If we can determine the absorbed dose in one material, such as air, we can convert this to the absorbed dose in another material such as water by multiplying by the ratio of their respective mass energy absorption coefficients. In section 5.2.2 we showed that dose to air is equal to air kerma when we have CPE. So we have now related exposure to air kerma to dose to air. Therefore, to convert dose to air to dose to water we use the equation below:

$$D_{water} = D_{air} \cdot (\mu_{en}/\rho)_{water}/(\mu_{en}/\rho)_{air}$$

For materials (media) with similar atomic number to air the ratio $(\mu_{en}/\rho)_{med}/(\mu_{en}/\rho)_{air}$ varies gradually and by not very much with energy. For water and air this ratio is approximately 1.1 between photon energies of 100 keV and 10 MeV. This is very fortunate as the distribution of photon energies (spectrum) does not need to be known precisely in order to accurately determine absorbed dose to water from a measurement of exposure.

For materials that have a higher atomic number than air, such as bone, the ratio can vary dramatically with energy (Figure 5.3). At lower energies the photoelectric effect is more probable in higher atomic number materials (proportional to Z^3) than in air and so the ratio of relative absorption will be large. As the energy increases into the Compton region, electron density becomes the important parameter in determining the interaction probability, making the ratio approximately constant. We can also see from this that at low energies bone can absorb over four times the energy per unit mass than water. For this reason, electron beams, which do not exhibit such differential absorption, may be favoured in such treatment cases.

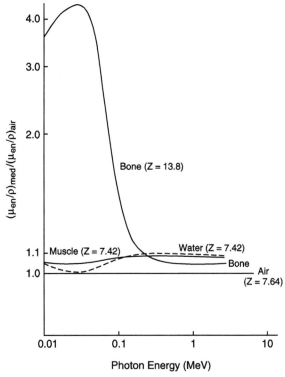

Figure 5.3 Variation of $(\mu_{en}/\rho)_{med}/(\mu_{en}/\rho)_{air}$ with photon energy.
Adapted with permission from Meredith and Massey, *The Fundamental Physics of Radiology*, 3rd Edition, J Wright 1977.

5.4 **Methods of radiation measurement**

5.4.1 Requirements of a dosimeter

Radiation produces several effects and quantifying an effect can give us a measure of dose. In principle, any effect could be used as the basis for dose measurement as long as the relationship between the measured effect and absorbed dose can be determined.

To perform well, a detector would fulfil a number of requirements. It would be sufficiently accurate across the range of doses be precise and sensitive. It would also be linear across the dose range used and independent of dose rate; have a response which is independent of dose (to measure large or small doses equally well). The response should be independent of energy and be able to represent dose in tissue and not just the material of the detector. Finally, it should be small enough to have spatial resolution for used in high dose gradients.

No detector fulfils all these requirements and different detectors are chosen for different measurement situations.

5.5 **Ionization chamber devices**

5.5.1 **Ionization**

If sufficient energy is transferred in an interaction of radiation with matter, ion pairs are formed. This ionization is caused by an electron absorbing sufficient energy that its energy then exceeds the binding energy of its atom and becomes free. It leaves behind a positively charged atom resulting in an ion pair. The amount of ionization produced is proportional to the energy delivered to the medium and so measurement of the amount of ionization can be the basis of not only a radiation detector but also of dose measurement. Ionization chambers usually measure charge created in air.

5.5.2 **Principles of operation**

5.5.2.1 The need for applied voltage

In order to measure the number of ions produced, they must be collected. This is done simply by attracting them to an electrode of opposite charge and counting them in a device called an electrometer. In travelling through the medium, the ions produced will be attracted to any ions of opposite charge in the vicinity and there will be a tendency to recombine. If recombination occurs the ionization event cannot be detected and hence will not contribute to the measurement and the dose will be underestimated. To minimize the chance of recombination, the potential difference (voltage) between the electrodes must be sufficient to collect the electrons quickly. The collection of electrons constitutes a current through the electrometer which can be measured by a current meter. As the voltage is increased, the number of electrons collected (i.e. prevented from recombining) increases until all of the available electrons are being collected. Leakage of charge collected from the chamber assembly must be minimized by using appropriate insulation materials.

5.5.3 **Types of ionization chambers**

5.5.3.1 Free air ionization chamber

The free air chamber is a primary standard designed to determine exposure for photon energies up to around 300 kV. Free air chambers are maintained by national standards laboratories and used to calibrate reference standards, which in turn are used to calibrate the routine equipment used in radiotherapy departments (see section 5.9). The free air chamber is designed to comply as closely as possible with the definition of exposure and the conditions to satisfy charge particle equilibrium and is shown schematically in Figure 5.4. It consists of an air-filled metal box with an aperture allowing a well-defined area (A) of X-rays to pass through the chamber so that it only interacts with air within the chamber. Ions created when the X-rays interact with the air are attracted toward two high voltage electrodes placed on opposite sides of the box. The electrode separation is sufficient to ensure that electrons emanating in the shaded region lose all their energy before they reach the electrodes, that is they are completely stopped in air. Electronic equilibrium is established as long as the shaded volume is sufficiently far inside the box that full electron build up has been achieved. This means that electrons produced in but travelling out of the dotted region and not collected by the electrodes are compensated for by electrons entering this region from outside and subsequently collected by the electrodes. The total electron charge (Q) is measured and the mass of air calculated from the air density (ρ) and dimensions of the shaded volume. Several small correction factors are applied to account for such things as X-ray attenuation in air between the entrance aperture and shaded collection region, the presence of any water vapour, scattered radiation entering the chamber from outside, ionization from bremsstrahlung, not all electrons being collected by the positive electrode, etc. For higher energies, although basic construction is similar, the NPL medium energy free air chamber (Table 5.1) capable of measuring energies in the range 40–300 kVp is substantially larger ($\sim 10^5$ larger sensitive volume) than its lower energy equivalent (8–50 kVp). This is necessary to satisfy the definition of exposure and to ensure electronic equilibrium is reached at the measurement volume.

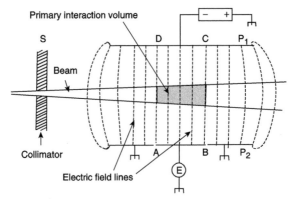

Figure 5.4 Schematic diagram of a free air ionization chamber. The guard plates outside the AB plate exclude any signal from the region where the electric field lines are bowed to ensure that the volume from which ionization is collected is known.

As the beam energy increases, the separation of the plates must also increase to prevent electrons reaching the plate before giving up all of their energy.

5.5.3.2 Thimble chambers

More useful in the radiotherapy department is a relatively small ionization chamber, usually thimble shaped, which encompasses a typically 0.1 cm^3 to 1.0 cm^3 cavity within which ionization occurs (the active volume) and is collected between the chamber's axial electrode and its conducting walls (see Figure 5.5). The walls are close to tissue or air equivalence using a low-Z material such as graphite or conducting plastic. The

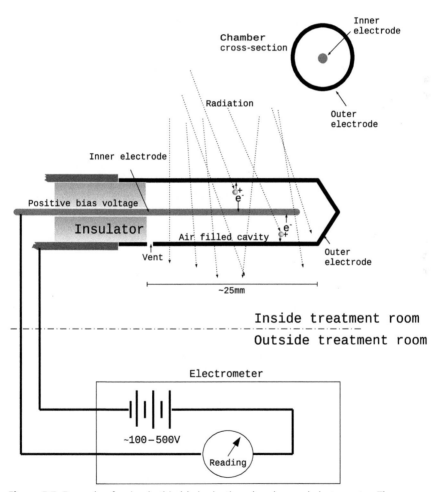

Figure 5.5 Example of a simple thimble ionization chamber and electrometer. The conducting inner and outer electrodes of the chamber are separated by an insulator. The chamber is connected to the electrometer outside the treatment room by a long cable which supplies the required voltage difference to the electrodes as well as conducting the small current produced from ionization in the air cavity. The guard ring reduces leakage through the insulator.

central electrode is usually aluminium. This has a high atomic number, but the effective atomic number of the detector as a whole is similar to air. The commonly used 'Farmer' -type thimble chamber has an external diameter of 7 mm, a 1 mm aluminium electrode, and a 0.5 mm graphite external wall making the gap between the electrodes 2.5 mm. In practice 200 V is used to guarantee collection of virtually all ions created. The thimble is one of the key components in a dosimetry system as it accurately defines the cavity volume in which ionization of the contained air mass occurs as well as forming one of the electrodes. The material the thimble is made from is important in determining the properties of the chamber. The standard Farmer-type cavity chamber is useable across the full range of radiotherapy energies from around 50 kV to 25 MV.

The theoretical basis on which the cavity type chamber can be used in the kV energy range (to 300 kV) is quite distinct to that in the MV energy range. At kV energies the thimble material is assumed to be air equivalent, whereas in the MV energy range it is assumed to be water equivalent. A detailed description is beyond the scope of this chapter, but a brief overview is given as follows for completeness.

For the free air chamber described above, if it were possible to compress the air around the shaded measurement volume (so that electronic equilibrium still holds) by, say, a factor of 1000 without affecting the shaded volume, the electron ranges in this compressed volume would also be reduced by a factor of 1000. If the electron fluence, that is the number, direction, and energy of electrons leaving this compressed volume were identical to that in air then the conditions of charged particle equilibrium would be satisfied. That is, if we could make a thimble out of compressed, solid, air, it would behave the same as the free air chamber. Suitable thimble materials (graphite, conducting nylon) having similar properties to 'very dense' air enable exposure measurement by simulating a free air chamber.

5.5.3.3 Parallel plate chambers

One disadvantage of the cylindrical thimble chamber is its inability to pinpoint the position of a dose measurement in a high dose gradient radiation field. Plane parallel (or parallel plate) chambers allow the measuring point to be much better defined in space and to have a finer measurement resolution in one dimension. A parallel plate chamber consists of two conducting plate walls, only one of which usually is the beam entrance wall as shown in Figure 5.6. Parallel plate chambers are recommended for measurements in electron beams and surface and build up dose measurements in photon beams.

5.5.4 **Electrometer**

5.5.4.1 Principles of operation

In order to convert ionization produced in a chamber into an indication of exposure, the ionization must be collected and measured. To quantify the rate of exposure, the rate of flow of charge (i.e. current) through the circuit should be measured with an ammeter. To quantify the total exposure, all of the charge produced in the cavity (which, when moving, constitutes the current) needs to be collected and measured. This is done by storing the charge in a capacitor until the end of the exposure and then

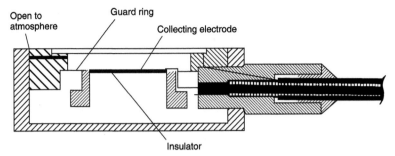

Figure 5.6 Plane parallel chambers. The measuring point is typically immediately inside the upper front face electrode. The guard ring defines the collecting volume.

reading the potential difference across it. The current produced by a 0.6 cm³ ionization chamber is typically 10^{-9}A or, for small volume pinpoint ionization chambers, as low as 10^{-12}A (a million millionth of an Amp). Electrometers may also be used to assess dose rate, rather than dose by measuring how the current change from moment to moment.

5.6 Other measurement devices

5.6.1 Solid state detectors

Detectors based on solid materials have a great advantage over gas-filled detectors. Their density is significantly greater than air and therefore their ability to cause inter-actions with incident radiation is much greater. The section below summarizes the most used solid state detectors.

5.6.1.1 Thermoluminescent detectors

If the light output from thermoluminescent (TL) materials can be measured and the amount of light produced is calibrated against absorbed dose then the TL material can be used as a dosimeter (TLD). Commonly used TL materials are lithium fluoride (LiF), which has an effective atomic number (8.2) close to that of tissue (7.4), and lithium borate ($Li_2B_4O_7$) with effective atomic number (7.3).

In single atoms, electrons can exist only in discrete energy states but the closely packed atomic structure of crystals means that interactions between adjacent atoms results in different bands of allowed energies: a lower range of allowed energies termed the valence band and an upper range termed the conduction band. The en-ergy range between, termed the forbidden region, is not available to electrons unless some impurity defines an energy state that electrons can hold. These intermediate energy states are called electron traps. In the case of LiF crystals, these traps can be created by the introduction of a tiny amount of manganese impurity atoms into the crystal structure.

When an electron in an atom absorbs energy from irradiation it may have its energy state raised from the **valence** band to the **conduction** band of energies. The electron may recombine with a positive 'hole' and return to its default 'ground' state emitting

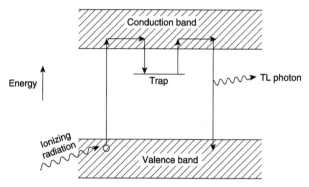

Figure 5.7 Energy level model of thermoluminescence process.

a photon of light in the process, resulting in the phenomenon called fluorescence. If an electron settles in one of the intermediate electron traps it is in a metastable state where energy is required to lift it out of its energy trap in order to return to its ground state, emitting a photon in doing so. In thermoluminescence, heat is be used to provide the required energy. This process is shown schematically in Figure 5.7 Electrons can reside in trap states for some time and this means that we can store a record of radiation exposure and later read them via thermoluminescence.

As the temperature applied is increased, the likelihood of releasing the trapped electrons increases and so the amount of light given off increases. If the crystal contains traps of different energies, then different amounts of heat are required to induce the emission of TL photon from each. The amount of light given off as a function of temperature when heat is applied shows a non-linear variation and is called a **glow curve** (Figure 5.8), which may contain a number of peaks associated with the different energy traps. The total light emitted is equivalent to the area under the glow curve and this can be calibrated with dose to produce a TL dosimeter. For a large range of radiotherapy energies, the light output is a linear function of dose. Before use, any existing (or residual from a previous exposure) trapped electrons (and holes) must be removed. This can be done using a heating and cooling cycle using specific temperatures and rates, a process called annealing.

TL dosimeters are useful for *in-vivo* measurements because they are small, for example 3 mm square × 1 mm thick, and do not require connection to measuring equipment with wires. Their main drawback is that their accuracy is limited to typically 3–5%. The dose response of TLDs is dependent on their anneal history and so batches of TLD chips should have the same anneal history.

5.6.1.2 Silicon diode detectors

A diode dosimeter consists of a silicon (Si) crystal with two regions; a p-region with an excess of positive charge (or deficit of electrons leaving positively charged 'holes') and an n-region with an excess of negative charge (electrons). In practice this is produced by taking a p-type Si substrate and introducing atoms of another material in a process called doping. This creates a region where p- and n-type Si are

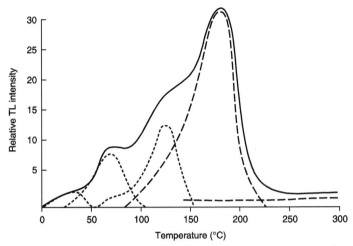

Figure 5.8 Glow curves and dose curve used for thermoluminescent dosimetry.

in direct contact. At this junction, local diffusion of electrons causes some of the holes in the p-region adjacent to the junction to be filled with electrons from the n-region. This results in a p-n junction region which is depleted of mobile charges and termed the depletion layer. Due to the diffusion of charges in this region a small intrinsic potential difference (~0.7 V) is created across this depletion layer. Free electrons generated by ionizing radiation within or sufficiently close to this p-n region such that they diffuse (from the p-side) into the depletion layer, will be swept across to the n-region, generating a current. This current can be measured in an electrometer without the need for an applied bias voltage. The active volume of the diode detector is therefore very small in this direction (≈100 μm). The diameter of the diode itself is of the order of 1–2 mm, encapsulated in waterproof material and, depending on use, added build up material making their outside dimensions typically from 3 mm to 10 mm.

The higher density of Si compared to air and the low average energy required to form an ion pair (~1/10th of that in air) results in a generated radiation current which is about 18,000 times that of air for the same measurement volume. The signal from a very small volume diode detector is therefore as great as a much larger air ionization chamber. The higher resolution afforded by these small volume detectors makes them particularly useful in measuring beam profiles (see section 6.4.1.2) because they can accurately measure the rapidly changing dose in the penumbra region. The sensitivity and resolution advantages are not enough to make a diode the ideal detector. One disadvantage is a change in sensitivity with repeated use due to radiation damage. This means that they should not be used for reference or absolute dosimetry (section 5.7). Even for relative dosimetry they need to be calibrated at a frequency consistent with the observed rate of sensitivity change. Modern diodes are often pre-irradiated to a large dose (kGy) which, although reducing their initial sensitivity due to radiation damage, makes their subsequent change in sensitivity with accumulated dose less pronounced.

Diodes are often used to check patient entrance doses and are produced with build-up material which is energy specific. Diodes exhibit a response variation with temperature, beam energy spectrum, dose rate, and angle of incidence and so careful use is required to get good performance. Temperature variation may be particularly difficult to deal with if the temperature of the diode is lower than the patient's skin when placed and increases in temperature during the exposure. Ideally the diode should be at the skin temperature at the point of measurement as well as calibration. Currently available commercial diodes exhibit relatively low sensitivity variation with temperature (typically only 1–2% increase in response between room and skin temperature (around 32 °C)).

5.6.1.3 MOSFET detectors

Metal oxide semiconductor field effect transistor (MOSFET) detectors are very small detectors with high spatial resolution. Because of their size they cause very little attenuation of the beam. Ionizing radiation causes electrons to be permanently trapped in the oxide layer which results in a change in the threshold voltage of the transistor. A reader connected to the detector determines this change in threshold voltage and can convert this directly to dose if the detector has been suitably calibrated against a known dose. Because of the permanence of the trapped electrons, MOSFETs have a limited life as a dosimeter. They are often used to measure doses directly on patients but must be discarded after receiving typically 100 Gy which, depending on the treatment, could be only a few patients' use.

MOSFETs do not require a dose rate correction but they do have a small variation in response with energy. Like diodes, MOSFETs have a temperature dependence.

5.6.2 Chemical detectors

Radiation can cause chemical changes in some materials which, if calibrated, can be used in radiation measurement systems. The most commonly used material is radiographic film, historically used for diagnostic X-ray and radiotherapy dosimetry. However, because of the cost and need for chemical processing, radiographic film is seldom used and has largely been replaced by radiochromic film.

5.6.2.1 Radiochromic film

Radiochromic film, as the name suggests, changes colour upon exposure to radiation. The greater the exposure to ionizing radiation the greater the resultant colour density and the less light transmission it allows. It is a self-developing film and the colour change is caused by polymerization of dyes embedded in an emulsion layer coated on a substrate. Once produced, the polymer absorbs light.

The spatially variant opacity allows the original exposure variation to be viewed by shining a uniformly illuminated light through the film. For dosimetry, light transmission is measured, using an optical densitometer, in terms of optical density which is a logarithmic function of the light intensity measured with (I) and without (I_0) the film at the position of measurement. Optical density (OD) is defined as $\log_{10}(I_0/I)$. The absorption peak depends on the film type used and the best contrast will be achieved if wavelengths around this region can be extracted. The useful dose range of the currently available film is in the region 0.01 Gy–20 Gy. Although the film does not require chemical development, the post exposure dose image continues to develop over time and it should be left for typically 6 hours to stabilize before readout.

Radiochromic film has many advantages:

1) High spatial resolution.
2) No dark room required, but the film needs to be kept away from light.
3) Response independent of dose rate.
4) Nearly tissue equivalent.
5) Can be submerged in water

The disadvantage is:

1) Non-linearity of response.

To achieve accuracy in the range of 3%, radiochromic film still requires a carefully setup and well-maintained scanning and processing system and dose calibration process.

5.7 **Detectors for dose measurement**

5.7.1 **Absolute dosimetry**

Absolute dosimetry refers to the direct measurement of dose and is seldom performed outside standards laboratories. For kV energies, a free air chamber is used but for megavoltage energies it is most often based on measurement of temperature rise in a graphite calorimeter. The temperature rise is tiny (pico degrees) and is only measurable with specialist equipment.

5.7.2 **Reference dosimetry**

Reference dosimetry is the determination of absorbed dose using a well-defined standard setup and using approved reference standard electrometer and ionization chamber which is cross calibrated against a primary standard. In the United Kingdom, the approved secondary standards, known as designated transfer instruments, are all ionization chambers that demonstrate a high standard of stability with respect to variations in energy, dose, and dose rate. The chambers used for external beam photons are typically Farmer type, with parallel plate-type chambers for electrons and well type for brachytherapy sources.

5.7.3 **Relative dosimetry**

There are many dose measuring devices that do not fulfil the stringent requirements of reference dosimetry. These can still be very useful in situations where we are interested in how dose changes rather than actual dose measurements. These measurements are useful if the same corrections would be appropriate for both measurements. In this case it is unnecessary to make the ionization to dose corrections, and indeed, the required corrections may not be known. Examples of such measurements are depth dose measurements such as percentage depth doses, or field size factors, both discussed in Chapter 6. In choosing a device for relative dosimetry it must be known what quantities are changing between the relative measurements and a device which is insensitive to this change can be selected.

5.8 Relationship between ionization and dose

5.8.1 Phantom materials

The reference material for performing dosimetry measurements is either water or a water-equivalent material. A water-equivalent material is designed to have the same radiation interaction characteristics as real water over the energy spectrum at which the measurements will be made. Commercial solid water-equivalent plastic materials consist of a homogenous mixture of several materials combined in appropriate proportions to produce an accurate match with water. These may also include materials to modify the density to that of water so that depths in the water-equivalent material match those in real water. The advantage of water-equivalent materials is that although a lot more expensive than real water, they are rugged and enable quick, easily reproducible, and accurate setup.

5.8.2 Dose measurement in the Radiotherapy Department

At MV energies, electron ranges in the irradiated material are much greater than at kV energies and even the 'very dense' air thimble would have to become thick to provide electronic equilibrium leading to unwanted attenuation of the photon beam. At these energies a theoretical approach called Bragg–Gray cavity theory is adopted. First, we need to imagine a small air-filled cavity introduced into a material uniformly irradiated by photons in which charged particle equilibrium exists. If the introduction of this cavity does not modify the electrons in any way, then the electron fluence passing through the air in the cavity would be the same as in the material in the absence of the cavity. If the same number and energy of electrons pass through the material and air cavity then the ratio of electron energy lost per unit mass equals the ratio of the mass stopping powers of the material and gas concerned. So by measuring exposure and deriving the dose to air we can then calculate the dose to the surrounding material by multiplying by the ratio of the mass stopping powers for the material, usually water, and air.

5.9 Calibration and traceability of dose determination

5.9.1 The calibration chain

The first requirement of all dosemeters is that they exhibit some response (R) to radiation. To use that response as a measure of dose requires an additional factor, the calibration factor (F) that under the conditions in which the device was irradiated will convert the response to absorbed dose (D).

$$D = F \times R$$

For equipment used in the clinic this factor is routinely determined by comparing the uncalibrated device with another device that is already calibrated. The calibration factor is then the multiplier required to make the uncalibrated reading match the known dose as shown by the calibrated device.

This process of determining the calibration factor for a new device is called an intercomparison or cross calibration. This process must be performed with care. Dosimetry Codes of Practice (CoP) describe in detail how this is carried out. CoPs provide definitive guidance on:

1) Performing a cross calibration between a calibrated secondary standard and an uncalibrated dosemeter;

2) Conducting an absorbed dose measurement using a calibrated dosemeter.

At the top of this calibration 'chain' sits a device that cannot be calibrated by comparing with another. The calibration chain starts with a primary standard, a device that determines the quantity of interest from first principles. In this hierarchy all devices depend on the accuracy of the primary standard. Figure 5.9 shows this calibration chain from the centrally maintained primary standard down into the hospital clinic. Each vertical arrow indicates that a cross-calibration must take place in order to propagate the primary standard calibration down the chain. The CoP details how absorbed dose is to be measured in the clinic and how the cross-calibration between secondary standard and routine equipment is performed.

5.9.2 Dose standards

5.9.2.1 National standards

By their nature, primary standards are complex pieces of equipment requiring dedicated full-time staff for maintenance and operation. These standards are not transportable and are inappropriate for use in a clinical setting. They are maintained at a national level in dedicated primary standard dosimetry laboratories (PSDLs). In the United Kingdom this is the National Physical Laboratory (NPL) at Teddington,

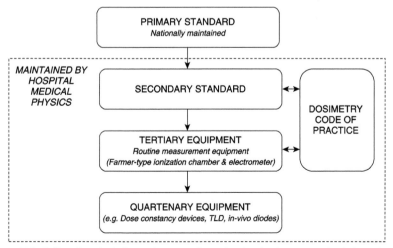

Figure 5.9 Calibration chain from the centrally maintained primary standard down into the hospital clinic.

Table 5.1 Four primary standards covering external beam photon and electron radiotherapy

Primary standard	Energy range	Quantity realized
Free in air	8.5–50 kVp	Air kerma
Free in air	50–280 kVp	Air kerma
Graphite calorimeter (photons)	Co60–25 MV	Absorbed dose to water
Graphite calorimeter (electrons)	4–20 MeV	Absorbed dose to water

Middlesex. There are currently five primary standards covering external beam photon and electron radiotherapy maintained at NPL and these are summarized in Table 5.1.

To satisfy the conditions of charged particle equilibrium, the size of a free air chamber should be around twice the range of the maximum energy electrons generated from the photons being measured. At higher energies this becomes impractical as it would require a chamber several metres across. As a result, standards laboratories use air-filled graphite-walled cavity ionization chambers to realize air kerma at higher energies. Graphite is reasonably air equivalent but has a much higher density and therefore can be thought of as a large volume of air compressed into a much thinner rind of graphite. It relies on the fact that the volume of the air cavity within the graphite is accurately determined. For a known volume and atmospheric conditions the precise mass of air inside the small cavity can be calculated. The charge liberated by this known mass of air can then be used to calculate the dose to air. Air kerma can then be derived from this dose to air using additional factors and Bragg–Gray cavity theory.

Charges liberated in a medium by ionizing particles result in an energy cascade in which energy is shared amongst many secondary particles. Eventually these less energetic charges and ions recombine with the resultant energy being liberated as heat. Although the number of ionizations generated per treatment fraction is sufficient to cause cell death, the energy involved is very small. Calorimetry is the technique of deriving absorbed dose via a measurement of temperature rise. The principle of calorimetry is straightforward, but the practical realization is difficult due to the small temperature rises involved. The absorbed dose in an irradiated medium is given by the measured temperature rise multiplied by the specific heat capacity of the medium. The specific heat capacity is the energy required per unit mass of material to increase its temperature by 1 °C.

$$D_{med} = C_{med} \times \Delta T$$

where:

D_{med} = Absorbed dose to the medium (J kg^{-1})

C_{med} = Specific heat capacity of the medium (J kg^{-1}°C^{-1})

ΔT = Temperature rise (°C)

The assumption in the equation above is that no other physical or chemical changes occur in the irradiated material that may result in absorbed energy not being manifested as a rise in temperature. Graphite is currently used for primary standard calorimeters. Compared to water it is a rugged stable material with a temperature rise six times that of water for the same dose (0.0014 °C/Gy for graphite). The downside of using graphite is that the measured dose is to graphite and must be converted to that in water.

Compatibility of measurements in different countries depends on the consistency of their respective national standards. This is tested by comparing primary standards directly or via an intermediary, such as the International Bureau of Weights and Measures (BIPM) in Paris, who coordinates the international measurement system. Internationally there are currently four different methods in use for establishing absorbed dose to water and these display a remarkable agreement (< 1%). There are currently four primary standards covering external beam photon and electron radiotherapy maintained at NPL and these are summarized in Table 5.1.

5.9.2.2 Local standards

The role of the PSDLs is to provide a calibration factor for the local (or secondary) standard. The term 'secondary' is used to denote it is calibrated against the primary standard. This local standard is maintained by one or perhaps a group of several hospital radiotherapy-physics departments and sent to the primary standards laboratory typically every three years for recalibration. The local standard is normally only used to cross-calibrate other 'tertiary' equipment, typically annually, used for routine measurements. The main use of routine equipment is to calibrate the output from the treatment equipment and then to confirm machine stability over time by repeat measurements at fixed intervals. The term output means absorbed dose (Gy) per set machine monitor unit (or time for some equipment) under appropriate reference conditions. Additionally, tertiary equipment will be used to calibrate other quaternary equipment such as dose constancy check devices, *in-vivo* diodes, TLD, etc. Secondary standard equipment is built to a higher quality and performance specification than equipment used for routine measurements and requires careful maintenance so that its calibration factors remain valid over the periods between subsequent recalibration at the PSDL.

5.9.3 **Dose measurement corrections**

The equation $D = F \times R$ described above to determine the dose (D) based on a dosemeter response (R) and calibration factor (F) strictly requires the dosemeter to be subsequently used under identical conditions at which it was calibrated for the calibration factor to be valid. Possible variations in conditions are many and some are listed below:

1) Temperature

2) Pressure

3) Humidity

4) Detector orientation

5) Depth of measurement

6) Total dose delivered

7) Dose rate (dose per linear accelerator (linac) pulse)

The less sensitive a detector is to any of the above the better. However, all detectors are sensitive to one or more of the variations listed. This means that the response of the detector must be corrected to the conditions under which it was calibrated.

Chapter 6

X-ray beam physics

Ranald MacKay and Alan Hounsell

6.1 **X-ray beams used in clinical practice**

In external beam radiotherapy, the radiation originates in a machine some distance from the patient surface. X-rays are only produced when the 'beam is on' and are the result of the collision of accelerated electrons with a target material; thus, X-rays are bremsstrahlung radiation (section 2.2.3). An important determinant of beam energy is the electrical potential through which a beam is accelerated. When an electron is accelerated across a voltage of 50,000 V it will acquire energy of 50,000 eV and this is the maximum energy that can be transferred to the X-ray produced by the bremsstrahlung interaction of the electron with a target. Often the energy on a treatment machine will be referred to by a kilovoltage (kV) or megavoltage (MV) potential that represents this maximum possible energy: most of the photons will have less energy than this maximum and the spectrum of energies of an X-ray source will have a peak at approximately one-third of the maximum (see Chapter 2, Figure 2.2).

The shape of the photon energy spectrum of the X-ray beam depends on the target material, filtration of the beam, and design of the X-ray head. However, the penetration of the beam is related to the maximum accelerating potential. X-ray treatment machines range from superficial X-ray units, designed only to treat to a depth of < 5 mm, to linear accelerators intending to treat tumours in the middle of the body (Table 6.1).

Although megavoltage strictly applies to any beam over 1 MV, in practice radiotherapy beams typically range from 4 MV to 25 MV with the most common combination for a standard accelerator delivering intensity modulated radiotherapy (IMRT) and volumetric modulated arc therapy (VMAT) to be a 6 MV and 10 MV dual photon energy.

6.2 **Beam quality and quality indices**

Beam quality is a measure of its ability to penetrate a material—the higher the energy the more penetrating the beam is (See Table 6.1). However, beams of the same energy produced on different machines may penetrate a material to different amounts. This is due to small differences in the energy of the accelerated electrons, the thickness and composition of the target, effect of any added filtration, and the design of the beam defining system.

Table 6.1 Range of use of different radiotherapy treatment units

	Accelerating potential	Clinical treatment depth	Clinical use
Superficial	50 kV–160 kV	< 5 mm	Skin lesions
Orthovoltage	160 kV–300 kV	< 6 cm	Shallow targets e.g. skin, superficial tissues, and ribs
Megavoltage	> 1 MV	< 30 cm	Deep seated tumours e.g. prostate

It is important to specify the energy of a beam for several reasons:

1) To be able to predict the penetrative characteristics of the beam;

2) For use with dosimetry protocols in which data from standard laboratories are specified in terms of energy (see Chapter 5);

3) To allow the comparison of treatments units and the outcomes of clinical studies between different centres (see Chapter 15). There are a number of ways of describing the beam quality and these are discussed next.

6.2.1 Quality indices for kilovoltage X-rays

The particular quality index used to describe a beam is dependent on the energy of that beam. At kV energies, the half value layer (HVL) (see Chapter 2) is used, that is the thickness of a specified absorber which reduces the beam intensity to half its original value. It describes the ability of the beam to penetrate a material and is therefore clinically relevant. The HVL is obtained by measurement of an absorption curve using the specified material. Sometimes beams of different spectral distributions can have the same first HVL but different second HVL values. This is due to the beam being comprised of a spectrum of X-ray energies which are differentially attenuated. The ratio of the first to second HVL is termed the homogeneity index and is 1 for a monoenergetic beam and less than 1 for heterogeneous beams. When measuring HVL the use of good geometry and the reduction of scattered radiation is important. When a broad beam is incident on sheets of attenuating material there is additional scattered radiation in addition to the primary radiation. This results in a seemingly more penetrating beam, the magnitude of that increase depending on the field size (Figure 6.1).

Kilovoltage and orthovoltage beams are specified in terms of their HVL, their peak kV value (kV_p) and often the filtration added to harden the beam before the HVL measurement is made. Example values are shown in Table 6.2. Superficial energy HVLs are usually specified in terms of millimetres (mm) of aluminium, higher energies being specified in terms of mm of copper.

6.2.2 Quality of megavoltage beams

HVL in pure metals (as used for kV beams) is not suitable at MV because it is both a slowly varying function of energy and it can be affected by pair production at higher

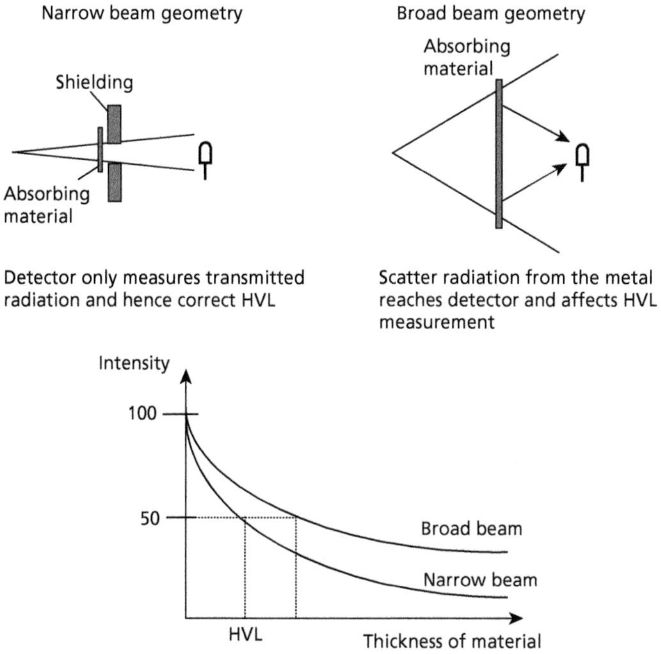

Figure 6.1 Correct narrow and incorrect broad beam geometries for measuring HVL and the resulting shape of the attenuation curves.

energies. Water is a more suitable material because it is tissue equivalent. There are several ways of using water to specify the energy of the beam.

6.2.2.1 Tissue phantom ratio (TPR_{10}^{20}) aka quality index (QI)

This specifies X-ray attenuation by measurement of the ratio of two points on a depth ionization curve well beyond d_{max}. This avoids any problems associated with measurements being made at d_{max} which can be influenced by electron contamination of the beam. The tissue phantom ratio (TPR) measurements use the ratio of the dose at two depths at a fixed source to detector distance. To characterize the energy, the ratio is used of the dose at 20 cm deep to 10 cm deep for a field size of 10 cm × 10 cm in water at a fixed chamber source distance of 100 cm (Figure 6.2).

Table 6.2 Nominal HVL values for typical kV values and added filtration values

kV$_p$	Typical added filtration values (mm Al)	Nominal HVL (mm Al)
100	1.15	2.1
70	0.75	1.1

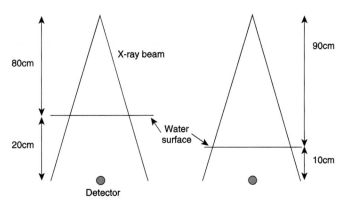

Figure 6.2 Measurement geometries for determining the QI at megavoltage energies.

The difference in dose is predominantly due to attenuation of the radiation in the water because both measurements are made at the same distance, which removes inverse square effects.

Although not strongly dependent on beam energy, this ratio is widely used to specify beam quality, especially for dosimetry purposes. For example, in the UK MV dosimetry chain (see Chapter 5) a hospital obtains calibration factors from the National Physical Laboratory (NPL) for its secondary standard dose meter by relating its local beam energies to beam energies measured at the NPL using the QI.

There are several other ways for specifying the beam energy.

6.2.2.2 Using percentage depth dose (PDD) data

The ratio of two central axis percentage depth dose values, measured at specific depths and for a specific field size can be used as a measure of the beam energy. The surface of the phantom is at a fixed source-to-surface distance (SSD), and field size is specified at the surface. This is commonly used for quality control measurements and is simple to perform but is not a very sensitive measure of energy. Typical depths used are 5 cm with 15 cm or 10 cm with 20 cm.

Another method is to use the PDD value at some distance beyond d_{max}. There are two ways of doing this:

1) the depth of a particular PDD value, for example d_{80}(cm);
2) the dose at a particular depth, for example D_{10}(%).

The advantages of these specifiers are that they are relatively easy to measure and vary significantly over the whole quality range and are usually at clinically relevant depths (Figure 6.3). Both these are used with linear accelerator (linac) manufactures often specifying the beam quality using the D_{10}(%) value.

The British Journal of Radiology (BJR) Supplement 25 provides detailed information about typical values for these metrics. Some example values are given in Table 6.3.

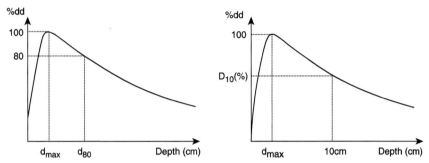

Figure 6.3 Schematic illustrating different methods for specifying energy of a beam using the PDD.

6.3 Depth dose characteristics

The dose deposited in a patient can be considered in three main parts (Figure 6.4):

- The surface dose;
- The build-up region;
- The region beyond the depth of maximum dose.

As a photon beam enters a medium it begins to lose energy through interactions with the atoms in the material. The dominant interactions for radiotherapy are the photoelectric effect, Compton scattering or pair production (section 2.4). The most common interaction at MV energies is Compton scattering, which produces predominantly forward scattered electrons that travel through the medium, ionizing atoms and depositing dose. The kinetic energy released from the photon beam to the electrons is known as kerma (kinetic energy release per unit mass—see section 5.2.2). Kerma is highest at the surface, where the photon beam has the greatest intensity, but paradoxically the dose is low. Kerma decreases with depth as the beam is attenuated, that is the number of photons available to transfer energy decreases.

There is some dose at the surface from radiation backscattered from the phantom, and contamination radiation (photons and predominantly electrons) from the treatment head and air gap. The surface dose value decreases with increasing energy. This reduces the dose to skin at the entrance of a radiotherapy beam, an effect called 'skin

Table 6.3 Example nominal values for different methods for specifying beam energy at MV energies

Nominal MV	$D_{10}(\%)$	$d_{80}(cm)$	d_{max}	QI	PDD(5)/PDD(15)
4	63.0	5.9	1.0	0.626	1.80
6	67.5	6.7	1.5	0.677	1.68
8	71.0	7.5	2.0	0.713	1.61
15	77.3	9.2	3.0	0.757	1.52

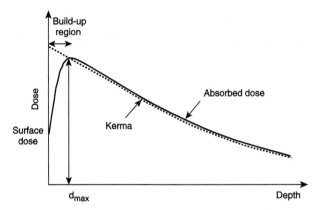

Figure 6.4 Dose (solid line) and kerma (dashed line) as a function of depth. The build-up region relates to the part of the curve before the dose reaches the maximum. At greater depths, the dose falls off due to the attenuation of the beam and also the spreading of the radiation from the source.

sparing'. Skin dose increases with increasing field size and if physical wedges are introduced into the beam. Practically, dose at the surface is difficult to measure because of the rapid gradient of the depth dose curve, the lack of electronic equilibrium, and the complexity of using standard ionization chambers which are designed to measure dose at depth.

Moving into the phantom, fewer photons are available to interact and the kerma falls but the dose is demonstrating 'build up' as the electrons set in motion at or close to the surface come to the end of their path and deposit more energy. At a depth below the surface, d_{max}, the dose reaches a maximum. At this point, in theory, the kerma curve intersects the dose curve and we have a point of charged particle equilibrium (CPE, see Chapter 5) where the energy deposited is the same as the energy transferred. In practice, the assumption generally is invalid due to the presence of contaminating electrons generated by the beam outside the phantom between the radiation source and the phantom surface. d_{max} increases with energy, it can also vary with field size and with the addition of physical wedges. This is due to additional contamination radiation contributing to the dose in the build-up region.

Beyond d_{max}, kerma and dose both decrease due to attenuation of the photon beam and the inverse square law. The rate at which the beam is attenuated depends on its energy—the higher the beam energy the less attenuation. However, the reduction in dose due to the beam spreading out is governed by the inverse square law which is **independent** of energy and is approximately 2% per cm at a distance of 100 cm. As kerma falls and less energy is transferred, less energy is deposited. Both curves decrease in parallel, the kerma curve being lower, separated by a distance dependent on the photon energy. The higher the energy, the greater the distance travelled by electrons set in motion before they come to the end of their path and deposit most dose. The relationship between kerma and dose beyond d_{max} is constant and transient charged particle equilibrium (TCPE) is said to exist.

6.3.1 Variation with field size

The PDD characteristics of a beam change with changes in field size as illustrated in Figure 6.5a. This is because the dose at depth in a material has a component due to scattered radiation. The amount of scattered radiation increases with increasing volume of material irradiated and this depends on surface field size and depth within the material. As the field size increases, the beam becomes more penetrating due to the increased scattered radiation. The magnitude of this effect is also energy dependent, being more pronounced for kV energies and less pronounced for MV energies. The reason for this is the direction of scatter produced. At lower energies, scatter occurs in all directions whereas at MV energies it is in the direction of the beam, so contributing relatively less dose to the central axis dose.

6.3.2 Variation with energy

The depth dose characteristics of a beam change with the beam energy. This is due to changes in the attenuation of the beam which is a function of beam energy. The higher the energy of the beam the more penetrating the beam as illustrated in Figure 6.5b.

6.3.3 Variation with focus-to-surface distance (FSD)

The PDD characteristic of a beam changes with FSD (Figure 6.5c). This is because the PDD contains both a component due to attenuation of the beam and an inverse square component. As the FSD increases the beam becomes more penetrating as the influence of the inverse square component reduces. Similarly, as the FSD decreases the beam becomes less penetrating as the inverse square component becomes more dominant. Note that for a given field size and energy, the surface dose is fairly constant once the FSD is 90 cm or more. If the FSD decreases below 90 cm, more electrons generated in the accelerator head can now reach the surface and the surface dose starts to increase.

6.4 Methods to describe the treatment beam

In this section definitions of beam geometry and field size are considered before the concepts around isodose lines are discussed.

6.4.1 Beam geometry

It is important to have a standard definition of beam geometry. As the beam is diverging, the treatment field will increase with increasing distance from the X-ray source.

6.4.1.1 Field size definition

This is a description of a square or rectangular field using two dimensions. The field size is usually defined at the isocentric plane which is typically at 100 cm FSD. The field size at the isocentric plane is also referred to as the jaw settings. Alternately the **surface** field size may be used which will differ from the jaw settings unless, of course, the surface is at the same distance as the isocentric plane. The field will diverge with increasing distance from the X-ray source and so treatments at extended or reduced FSDs will have a different surface field size than the accelerator jaw positions indicate.

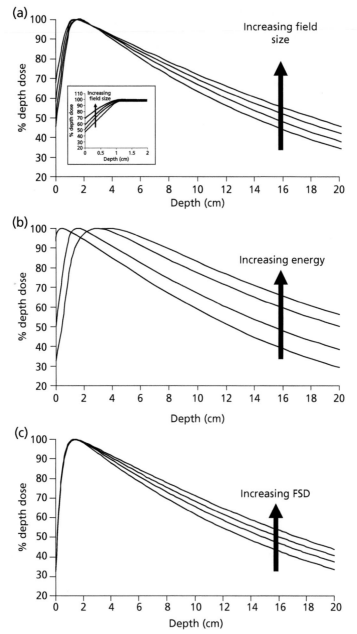

Figure 6.5 Variation of % depth dose with a) field size for square fields of sides 5, 10, 20, 40 cm at 6MV; b) with energy for Co-60, 6 MV, 15 MV, and 25 MV; c) with FSD for 80 cm, 100 cm 120 cm, and 150 cm for a 10 cm × 10 cm field at 6 MV.

Two definitions of field size can be used: the geometric field size and the dosimetric field size. The geometric field size is a projection of the front edges of the collimator system into the field by lines drawn from a point at the centre of the front face of the source. Such lines define the geometric edge of the beam. The dosimetric field size is the area enclosed by a specified isodose line. The geometric field size is equivalent to that defined by the 50% isodose while the therapeutically useful field size is usually defined by the 90% or 95% isodose lines. Care must be taken when considering fields less than 4 cm × 4 cm. When the collimator of the beam defines such a small field that the finite photon source is occluded, and there is a loss of lateral charged particle equilibrium, then the relationship between the geometric and dosimetric field size breaks down. Specific professional guidelines on small field dosimetry should be followed.

6.4.1.2 Beam profiles and penumbra

A beam profile is a plot of dose across the beam in a direction perpendicular to the central axis, passing through the central axis, and normalized to the dose at the central axis.

There are several key features of the beam profile that can be demonstrated by looking at a profile measured at 10 cm deep in water at the isocentre (Figure 6.6). The beam

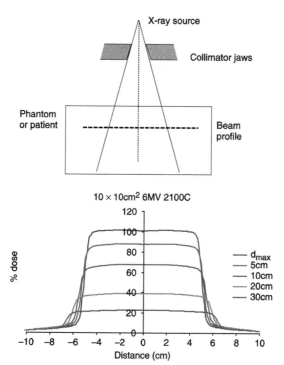

Figure 6.6 Schematic illustrating the measurement conditions and a series of beam profiles taken at different depths in the phantom.

profile is normalized to the intensity in the centre of the beam. Two important measurements that can be made from the profile are the flatness and the symmetry. The flatness is an expression of the difference between maximum dose and minimum dose across the beam profile at a defined depth in water in the central 80% of the beam. Beam flatness is characterized by a filter in a linac head (see Chapter 11). Beam symmetry is an expression of the dose at two points on a beam profile, each equidistant from the central axis. A beam is generally considered symmetric when these points are within 3% of each other but modern linacs usually produce beams well within this value. A flat and symmetric beam is desirable for radiotherapy planning; changes in flatness and symmetry may indicate changes in the beam energy or the steering of the beam in the wave guide. The flatness of the profile changes as a function of depth, field size, and beam energy.

The edge of the beam is known as the penumbra. This can be defined as the distance between the 80% and 20% dose at the isocentric plane at depth. The penumbra is due to the finite size of the X-ray source (Co-60 source, linear accelerator focal spot size) and scattered radiation; photons from the field and secondary electrons (released by photon interactions) out of the beam. The shape is affected by the focal spot size and shape (which can be elliptical, rather than circular), scattering of photons and electrons, and the shape and properties of the collimators (section 11.3.2.5). The penumbra is larger for the upper (inner) jaws than for the lower (outer) jaws. The extent of the penumbra changes with depth in the medium. Looking further outside the penumbra the dose tails off and is mainly due to scattered radiation from the open part of the beam and transmission though the jaws of the treatment unit.

Due to divergence, beam profiles become wider at deeper depths. In addition, there is more scattered radiation, so the penumbra becomes wider (Figure 6.7). As the beam is attenuated the intensity is reduced as indicated by the fall off in the depth dose curve.

6.4.2 Isodose lines

A line joining all points in a plane that have the same percentage dose value is called an **isodose line**.

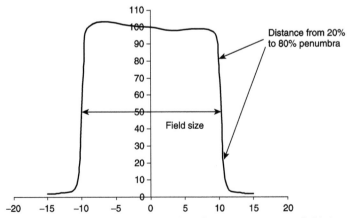

Figure 6.7 Beam profile measured at 10 cm deep for a 20 cm × 20 cm field size.

A chart showing a selection of isodose lines (usually in increments of 10% for a single beam) in any given plane is termed an isodose distribution. For superposed beams, fewer lines may be displayed for clarity.

6.5 **Beam-modifying devices**

The treatment beam can be both shaped geometrically and can have its intensity distribution modified. These can be achieved using IMRT techniques. Another widely used method for achieving simple changes in intensity is to use **wedges.**

6.5.1 **Principles of wedges**

Wedged beams are used for three main purposes:

1) Combining beams from non-orthogonal angles,

2) Compensating for changes in surface shape,

3) Compensating for changes in depth dose fall off for beams incident perpendicular to the wedged beam.

There are three types of systems that produce wedged beams:

1) Manual fixed physical wedges,

2) Universal physical wedge,

3) Dynamic wedges.

6.5.1.1 Manual or physical wedges

Physical wedges are rarely used nowadays. These are wedge shaped pieces of aluminium, brass, or steel. A series of different wedges is usually in use, for example 15, 30, 45, 60 degrees. These will have different physical dimensions and may be constructed of different materials. Inserting and removing the wedge can be difficult especially at non-zero gantry and collimator angles. Also carrying and storing them requires careful ergonomic design within the treatment room. They also block the light field used for setting up the patient, so the wedge is often inserted after the patient is set up, exacerbating the manual handling problems.

6.5.1.2 Universal physical wedge

A single physical wedge can be used to create a range of wedge angles by combining the wedge field with a plain or open field irradiation. This design of wedge is used in Elekta accelerators. The wedge is automatically positioned in the beam within the treatment head above the position of the mirror and below the monitor chamber. However, wedging can only occur in one direction which becomes a problem if the wedge is combined with a multileaf collimator (MLC), when being able to wedge both in the direction of the leaf movement and perpendicular to this may be useful.

6.5.1.3 Dynamic or virtual wedges

Dynamic or virtual wedges are created by moving a secondary collimator jaw across the treatment field while the beam is on. The amount of wedging is determined by the length of time the jaw is in the treatment field. Wedging in different directions can be achieved by movement of different jaws. For Varian dynamic wedges, the wedge factor is strongly dependent on field size and this effect needs to be carefully modelled within the treatment planning system. Off-axis and half-blocked wedged fields are created in the same way. Again, care is needed in modelling the wedge factor.

6.5.2 Wedge factor (WF)

To deliver the same radiation dose to a point within a wedged field as for a plain field the number of monitor units set on the accelerator needs to be increased. This is achieved by use of a WF. The WF is defined as the ratio of doses with and those without the wedge in place usually, but not always, at a point on the central axis of the beam:

$$\text{Wedge Factor}(\text{WF}) = \text{Wedged Field Dose/Plain Field Dose}$$

The reciprocal of the WF indicates the increase in monitor units (MUs) required to deliver the same dose as for an identical plain field. The WF is a function of wedge type, wedge angle, beam energy, field size and shape, off-axis position and depth (Figure 6.8).

6.5.2.1 WF variation with field size

For physical wedges, the WF increases with field size. This is due to the amount of scattered radiation from the wedge increasing as the field size increases, and is typically of the order of 5–10% for clinically useful field sizes. For dynamic wedges, the variation with field size can be much larger, up to 50% with increasing field size.

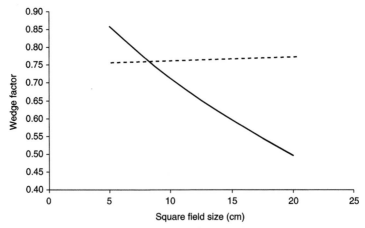

Figure 6.8 Wedge factor variation with square field size for a manual wedge (dashed line) and a Varian dynamic wedge (solid line) at 15 MV.

6.5.2.2 WF variation off-axis

Off-axis, the WF for physical wedges tends to follow the profile of the wedge i.e. they increase or decrease in the wedged direction and remain approximately constant in the non-wedged direction. For dynamic wedges, the WF approximately matches the on-axis factor for the same field size with only small differences being observed.

6.5.2.3 Effect on PDD

For physical wedges, the wedge hardens the beam i.e. increases the mean energy of the beam making the PDD for a wedged field more penetrating than for a plain field because the lower energy components of the photon spectrum are absorbed in the wedge. This is more pronounced at lower energies (4–6MV) where Compton scattering is predominant. At higher energies (>15MV), where pair production becomes more important, beam softening (a decrease of the depth dose with respect to the open field) is also possible. For dynamic wedges, there is no hardening of the beam and hence no change in the PDD or WF with changes in depth. The moving jaw attenuates the beams almost completely so there is no transmitted beam to harden.

6.5.3 **Wedge angle**

The wedge angle is defined as the slope of the line joining two points equidistant from the central axis and half the width of the field apart on the isodose curve which passes through the central axis at a reference depth (usually 10 cm). Alternate definitions include the angle between the tangent to a nominal isodose curve at the central axis, such as the 80% isodose curve, and the line perpendicular to the central axis (Figure 6.9). Wedge angles between 10 and 60 degrees are clinically used.

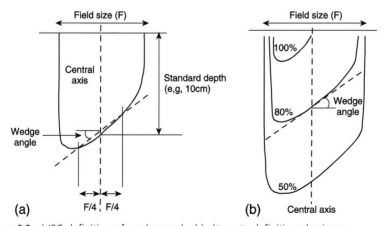

Figure 6.9 a) IEC definition of wedge angle; b) alternate definition also in use.

6.6 **Shaped fields**

This section considers the effects of shaped radiation fields. To understand how shaping a treatment field can affect the dosimetric characteristics of the beam it is helpful to consider the different components that contribute to the radiation dose for a radiation field.

6.6.1 **Primary dose**

This is the dose due to radiation incident on the phantom or patient (not scattered radiation from within the patient). It has two components: direct primary radiation and radiation scattered from within the treatment head (head scatter or sometimes termed collimator scatter).

6.6.1.1 Direct primary radiation

This component is radiation that has originated in the X-ray target and passes through the flattening filter without interacting. It is not dependent on field size.

6.6.1.2 Head scatter

This component is predominantly from radiation scattered from the flattening filter and from the collimator jaws, primary collimator, and monitor chamber and mirror. It is usually modelled as an extra focal source located at a scatter plane within the treatment head as shown in Figure 6.10a. This component is field size dependent; as the jaw size increases more of the scatter source is visible and hence more radiation emerges from the treatment head.

6.6.1.3 Collimator exchange

The head scatter component is responsible for the effect in which the output for an elongated field (e.g. 30 cm × 4 cm) is different from the output for the same elongated field with the longer field dimension changed between the jaws (e.g. 4 cm × 30 cm).

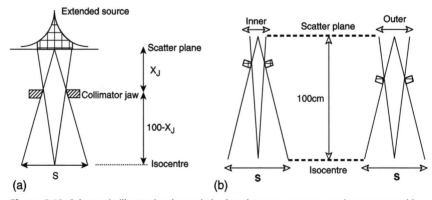

Figure 6.10 Schematic illustrating how a) the head scatter component is represented by an extended source and b) the location of the jaws within the treatment head affects the size of the extended source visible from the isocentre.

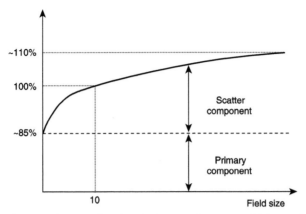

Figure 6.11 Schematic diagram showing the increase in output with increasing field size and how the relative contributions vary. Nominal values are shown which are indicative only.

This effect can be several percent and is due to the different jaws exposing different amounts of the scatter plane (Figure 6.10b). Even though the area of the extra focal source exposed by the two elongated fields remains the same, the shape is changed resulting in the different amounts of head scattered radiation.

6.6.2 Scatter in the patient

In the patient, radiation is scattered from the irradiated volume. This scattered radiation component is called the 'phantom scatter' component. The larger the surface field size the more scattered radiation there will be (Figure 6.11). The amount and proportion of scattered radiation will increase with increasing depth. Generally, there is more scattered radiation at lower energies.

6.6.3 Methods to account for scattered radiation

There are several ways in which changes in output with field size and shape due to scattered radiation are considered. The following deals with some more common methods.

6.6.3.1 Scatter factor (SF)

Scatter factor (SF) is defined as the ratio of the total absorbed dose at a point to the primary dose at that point:

$$SF = \frac{Total\,dose}{Primary\,dose}$$

SF depends on beam energy, field size and depth. SF goes to 1 as the field size goes to zero.

6.6.3.2 Peak scatter factor (PSF)

This is a special case of the scatter factor where the reference point is on the beam axis at the depth of maximum dose.

6.6.3.3 Backscatter factor (BSF)

This is a special case of the scatter factor where the point of interest is at the surface of the phantom. It is used at energies below 400 kV.

6.6.3.4 Output factor

The output factor is the dose at d_{max} for a set field size, normalized to a reference field size (usually a 10 cm × 10 cm field).

6.6.3.5 Tissue phantom ratio (TPR), tissue maximum ratio (TMR), tissue air ratio (TAR)

These quantities all give 'tissue dose' as a ratio of some reference dose which has been measured under reference conditions. To calculate the tissue dose you multiply the reference dose by the appropriate ratio. All these ratios refer to dose at the same point in the beam (i.e. at a fixed distance from the source), usually the isocentre. Hence there is no divergence and no SSD dependence. These ratios depend on depth (d), energy (E), and size and shape of the field. The depth dependence is due to attenuation and scattering and does not incorporate a divergence effect.

6.6.3.5.1 Tissue phantom ratio The TPR (Figure 6.2) is defined as the ratio of the absorbed dose at a point on the central axis at any given depth to the absorbed dose on the central axis at the same distance from the source but with the surface of the phantom moved so that the point is at a specified reference depth. The collimator settings remain unchanged.

6.6.3.5.2 Tissue maximum ratio TMR is a special case of the TPR in which the reference depth is the depth of maximum dose.

6.6.3.5.3 Tissue air ratio A TAR is defined as the product of the tissue maximum ratio (TMR) and the peak scatter factor (PSF). TARs were used for Co-60 units but have been replaced by TPRs for megavoltage calculations. TAR was originally defined as the ratio of the absorbed dose at a point on the central axis at a depth in tissue, to the tissue dose, in air at the same point in the beam. This leads to problems at higher energies where significant thicknesses of build-up material are required for electronic equilibrium and hence dose in air is not being measured. At high energies large build up thickness, as are required, give rise to attenuation and scattering, therefore the true primary dose is not being measured.

6.6.3.6 Equivalent square field

The depth dose characteristics of rectangular and circular fields can be represented by calculating an equivalent square field size with the same characteristics. This is not a square field of the same area but of a field whose dimensions can be represented by:

$$\sigma = \frac{2ab}{(a+b)}$$

where a and b are the two sides of the rectangle and σ is the dimension of one of the sides of the equivalent square. This is only an approximation. The BJR Supplement 25 has extensive tables of equivalent field sizes.

6.6.3.7 Scatter from irregularly shaped fields

For irregularly shaped fields, the Clarkson sector integration technique is often used. In this the irregular field is divided into a series of sectors of circular fields. These sectors can then be added to determine the output from the irregular field (see section 9.7.3). Dose calculations for irregularly shaped fields are usually undertaken within the treatment planning system.

Chapter 7

Electron beam physics

George Pitchford[†] and Andrew Nisbet

7.1 Electron beams used in clinical practice

High energy electron beams may offer advantages over those of photons. The shape of an electron beam depth dose curve is characterized by a small skin sparing effect, a relatively uniform dose for a definite depth around the depth of maximum dose (d_{max}), and a relatively steep fall off with a finite range. The anatomy of an individual PDD is shown Figure 7.1a and a representative set of central axis depth doses is shown in Figure 7.1b.

The primary aim of electron beam therapy is to offer a method of treating target volumes situated on the surface of a patient or extending below the surface to a limited depth. This can be useful where underlying tissue with a higher Z number, such as cartilage or bone, results in a higher absorbed dose due to an increase in photoelectric interactions when kilovoltage (kV) X-rays are used.

Historically electron beams were produced predominantly in the energy range 5–35 MeV. However, there is little advantage for electron beams compared to high energy photons at these higher electron energies and modern linear accelerators now provide high energy electrons in the energy range 4–20 Mega electron volt (MeV). There is increasing interest in the potential of very high energy electrons (VHEE, 50–250 MeV) as a therapeutic option, particularly for FLASH-radiotherapy involving ultrahigh dose rates (mean dose rate above 100 Gy/s).

Although the use of intensity modulated radiotherapy (IMRT) and volumetric modulated radiotherapy (VMAT) is now more common, in some instances electrons may still be used in several clinical settings:

♦ Skin and lips.

♦ Chest wall and neck, both after surgery and for recurrent disease.

♦ Boost doses to limited volumes.
   1. Tumour bed for breast—assumed gross tumour target volume (GTTV).
   2. Scar areas.

♦ Total skin irradiation for mycosis fungoides and cutaneous lymphomas.

Electrons have been used for many years to treat cutaneous basal and squamous cell carcinomas. Electrons have also been used with success in the management of Kaposi's sarcoma, although other treatment options are now largely employed.

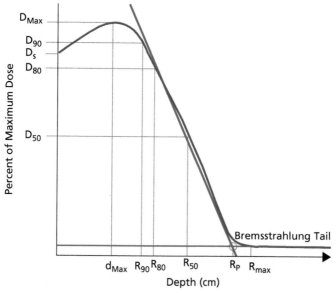

Figure 7.1a Showing the anatomy of an electron PDD and its range metrics. d_{max} is the depth of the maximum dose, in this case 100%. R_{90} and R_{50} are defined as the depth of the 90%, and 50% isodoses; D_{90} and D_{50} correspond to the percentage dose at these depths. R_p is the practical range of the electron beam, determined by extrapolation along the straight part of descending depth dose curve. R_{max} is the maximum depth of penetration of the beam after which dose is entirely due to bremsstrahlung X-rays created in the treatment head.

Reproduced with permission from International Atomic Energy Agency (IAEA), Strydom, W., Parker, W., Olivares, M., "Electron beams: physical and clinical aspects", Radiation Oncology Physics: A Handbook for Teachers and Students, IAEA, Vienna (2005) 273–300.

Post mastectomy patients can be treated with low energy electron beam radiation therapy, protecting underlying lung without sacrificing local disease control. Previously electron beams were used extensively in head and neck cancer, particularly when treating tissue overlying the spinal cord. Once photons had treated the region to a dose close to spinal cord tolerance, an electron field was used to boost the dose in this region while continuing to treat tissues away from the cord with photons. The relatively rapid fall off in dose at depth helps keep the dose to the spinal cord below tolerance. The electron and photon fields needed to be carefully matched. This technique, however, is now largely redundant due to intensity modulated radiotherapy.

Total skin electron therapy (TSET) is an effective treatment of mycosis fungoides, especially for patients who have thick generalized plaque or tumorous disease, and this technique may be used selectively for extra cutaneous disease. There are well defined dose response relationships for achieving a complete durable response. Electrons in the energy range 2–9 MeV are used given the rapid drop off in depth

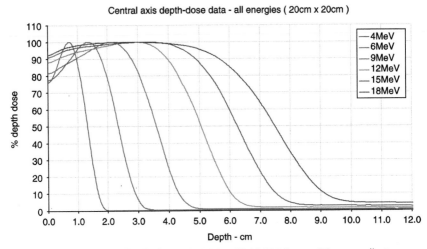

Figure 7.1b Central axis depth doses, 4 MeV to 18 MeV, 20 cm × 20 cm applicator.

dose and a low bremsstrahlung component. The bremsstrahlung tail (sometimes known as photon contamination) arises as the electron beam passes through the higher atomic number components of the treatment head. This enables superficial skin lesions to be treated to a depth of around 1 cm without exceeding bone marrow tolerance. A number of treatment techniques have been developed broadly based on either:

1) A translational methodology where the patient lies horizontally and is moved relative to a beam of sufficient width to cover the transverse direction of the patient.

2) A large field technique where a standing patient is treated with a combination of broad beams and extended SSDs (source-to-surface distance)

Although many of the treatments traditionally carried out by electrons are now done with IMRT/VMAT, electron beams will continue to have a role within radiotherapy for the foreseeable future. For example, some groups are exploring the use of intensity and energy-modulated electron beam radiotherapy which may be an option for shallow head and neck tumours. The use of dynamic mixed beam radiotherapy comprising intensity and energy modulated combined photon and electron beams is also being explored. This also been shown in retrospective planning studies to minimize heart dose in post mastectomy breast radiotherapy.

Most electron treatments are delivered as single fields with normal incidence at a fixed SSD, usually with an applicator present (see section 11.3.2.7). In some instances, the electron applicator is placed against the skin rather than with a fixed stand-off distance. Sometimes a non-standard SSD is required if the patient surface prevents positioning of the electron applicator at the standard SSD. Corrections to electron output for small changes in SSD may be needed. Strictly speaking, such corrections should use a modified inverse square law derived from a measured virtual source position.

7.2 **Energy ranges**

The interactions of electron beams are described in Chapter 3 and the concept of the continuous slowing down approximation (CSDA) introduced. The point at which the electron has lost all its energy identifies its range. If all electrons in the beam lose energy in the same way, all electrons will be stopped at the same depth. However, due to scattering, the actual depth reached will vary; this variation is known as range straggling. The path length (total distance travelled) will be the same for all electrons of the same energy (Figure 7.2). This explains the characteristic shape of an electron beam depth dose curve, with its high surface dose, relatively constant dose around the depth of maximum dose and then rapid drop in depth dose to a low dose tail arising from a bremsstrahlung X-ray component (Figure 7.1a). The electron range in cm can be approximated by dividing the mean electron energy in MeV by 2.

Depth doses in clinical data tables are usually presented in terms of the depth related to a specified percentage depth dose. When the oncologist has assessed the greatest depth of the relevant target volume then the energy required to effectively cover this volume can be read off the depth dose tables for that field size. Table 7.1 shows a selection of typical depth doses. However, be aware that these values are different for all linear accelerator (linac) types and local datasets for the real values for local treatment machines must be used in practice.

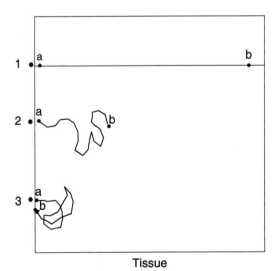

Tissue

Figure 7.2 Consider three electrons each travelling in tissue. They lose their energy, depositing it in tissue as dose, on their journey from a to b. The distance ab is the same for each, i.e. they have equal path lengths. However, the depth they reach in the tissue is very variable and depends on how scattered their path is. When applied to a huge number of electrons, the 'range' (depth in the tissue) will straggle over a set of distances; this is range straggle.

Table 7.1 Representative depths for a particular field size/applicator

Incident Energy (MeV)	6	8	10	12	14	16
Depth of maximum dose (cm)	1.2	1.8	2.3	2.9	3.3	3.7
Depth of 90%	1.7	2.3	3.1	3.9	4.7	5.2
Depth of 80%	1.9	2.7	3.5	4.3	5.1	5.6
Depth of 50%	2.3	3.0	4.0	4.9	5.8	6.4
Depth of 10%	3.0	3.9	5.2	6.0	7.3	8.3

The incident energy, E_0, is the mean energy at the surface of the patient. The practical range occurs at the intersection of dose fall off and the bremsstrahlung tail at about the depth of the 1–5% dose level and represents the range of the incident electron beam.

Of interest in assessing target coverage is the surface dose (see section 7.5), the depth of the maximum dose and the minimum tumour dose to be encompassed by the therapeutic range usually taken to be 90%, or occasionally 85%, isodose. The dose beyond the target is important to assessing dose to underlying, normal tissue.

7.3 Percentage depth dose

Referring again to Figure 7.1b, the depth dose curves have a number of properties:

- High surface dose which increases with energy (opposite to what happens for photon beams).
- Build up to the depth of maximum dose (which can be broad at high electron energies).
- Rapid dose fall off beyond dose maximum (higher energies give less rapid fall off).
- Low-value dose bremsstrahlung tail which increases slightly for higher energy beams.

There are a number of simple rules of thumb relating to central axis depth dose values:

- The therapeutic range 90% to 85% (on the fall off side of the curve) equals approximately one-third E_0 cm.
- Mean energy decreases by 2 MeV per cm in water or soft tissue and so the practical range, Rp, is 0.5 E_0 cm.
- The 50% depth dose lies halfway between the therapeutic range depth and the practical range depth. However, the depths of the 90% and 50% doses can be significantly reduced with small field sizes whilst the practical range remains unchanged (see section 7.4).

7.4 Factors affecting depth dose: field size

For field sizes larger than 10 cm × 10 cm, when the field size is changed, the central axis depth dose remains fairly constant beyond the build-up region. It does change within

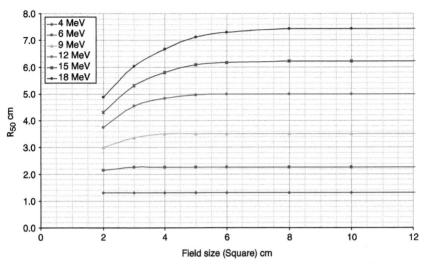

Figure 7.3 Effect of field size on R_{50} as a function of beam energy.

the build-up region. This is due to electrons scattering from the structure of the linear accelerator head, and the degree to which this occurs varies with the field size setting.

The consistency in central axis depth dose beyond d_{max} occurs when the distance from the central axis of the beam to the field edge exceeds the lateral range of scattered electrons, setting up an electronic equilibrium. This is particularly true for electron energies up to 10 MeV. This is demonstrated in Figures 7.3 and 7.4 which show respectively the variation of the depths of the 50% dose point (R_{50}) and d_{max} with field size and electron beam energy.

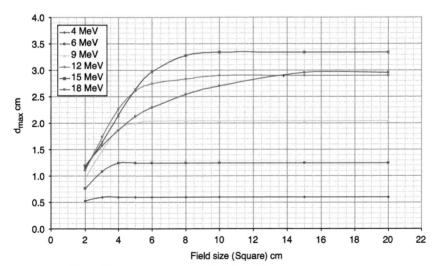

Figure 7.4 Effect of field size on d_{max} as a function of beam energy.

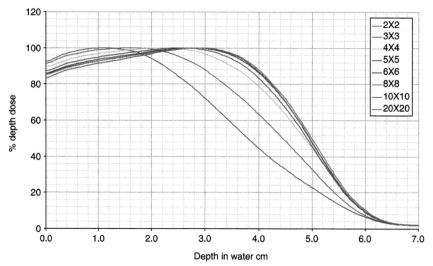

Figure 7.5 Effect of field size on depth dose for 12 MeV.

For energies above 14 MeV (according to accelerator design) it may be found that the position of the maximum (100%) central axis dose, d_{max}, may be closer to the surface at the highest energy than a lower E_0. This can be seen in Figure 7.1b for the 18 MeV curve.

For small field sizes, less than 6 cm square, the situation can be complicated. As the field gets smaller there is a loss of scattered electron equilibrium at the central axis of the field; this occurs even if only one of the dimensions falls below the practical range for the electron energy being used. The dose maximum and other high dose values are displaced towards the surface therefore increasing the surface dose. The practical range, which is dependent on the value of E_0, remains unchanged and hence the fall off gradient is reduced bringing a reduction in the therapeutic range. This is demonstrated in Figure 7.5.

Using a higher energy electron beam will not improve the therapeutic range because the higher the value of E_0, the more pronounced the effect of dragging the therapeutic range depth towards the surface. There is also a narrowing of the high dose isodoses (see section 7.6) that reduces the width of the volume encompassed by the therapeutic dose value. These effects need to be considered when prescribing small field electron treatments.

7.5 Build-up and skin sparing for electrons

The surface dose varies from approximately 75% to 95% depending on the initial electron energy. The dose increases with increasing energy as can be seen by the representative values in Table 7.2. There is only slight variation with field size with the caveat that small field sizes at high energies may behave differently.

Table 7.2 Electron surface doses, 6 MeV to 18 MeV, 6 cm to 25 cm applicators

Energy (MeV)	Electron Surface Doses Relative to 100% at Maximum Dose Applicator				
	6 cm	10 cm	15 cm	20 cm	25 cm
5	74.8	75.1	75.5	76.0	75.7
9	77.6	77.9	78.2	79.0	78.7
12	84.1	83.4	83.6	84.6	84.3
15	88.4	88.0	87.8	88.4	88.4
18	91.8	91.4	90.7	90.7	90.7

However, sometimes we do need a 90–100% dose at the surface, we can achieve this by using bolus. When doing this we will need to ensure the energy still is high enough to cover the deeper part of the volume.

Bolus is a flexible tissue equivalent material (e.g. Superflab™) which comes in a range of thicknesses. It is placed on the patient where the beam is to be directed. Wax can also be used as bolus and is often customized for each patient's treatment. The effect is to bring the high dose to the surface of the patient by allowing the dose build up to occur in the bolus itself. It may also be used to reduce the penetration of the beam in a particular part of the field to perhaps protect a vital organ lying behind the target volume, or to flatten out irregular surfaces such as those found in the head and neck region. The effect of bolus can be seen in Figure 7.6.

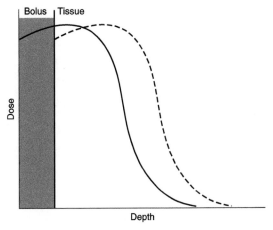

Figure 7.6 PDD curves for an electron beam with and without bolus.

7.6 **Isodose curves for electrons**

Electron isodoses are very different from the geometrical shape of a megavoltage photon beam. Since the electron beam energy is being constantly degraded as it penetrates through the patient, there is an increasing amount of laterally scattered electrons which results in an increasing penumbra with depth. As the electron beam passes through the patient it expands just past the surface of the patient, until a depth of where approximately 70% of the maximum dose is reached when it starts to narrow. Close to the surface the 50% isodose line follows the geometric field edge. The higher dose levels increase their separation from the 50% line and there is a constriction of the width of the high dose values which means that the high dose volume, above 90% is narrower at the therapeutic range depth than at the surface or d_{max}. These features can be seen in Figure 7.7. The constriction is approximately $2E_0$ mm on each side of the field and larger across a diagonal of a rectangular field. The value is accelerator dependent.

Lower dose levels bulge outwards so that at a depth there can be significant doses delivered outside the geometric edge of the field. This may need to be considered if there is a critical organ nearby the edge of the beam.

7.6.1 **Clinical aspects**

If the target volume is superficial then the energy selected to encompass the therapeutic range may not produce a sufficient surface dose. In this case, bolus or an energy degrader is used to increase the surface dose and a higher energy selected to maintain the required dose to the distal target volume. The field size may have to be a compromise between the need to have a wider beam at the patient's surface to encompass

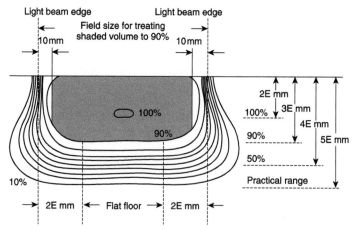

Figure 7.7 Electron isodose curve.
Reproduced with permission from *Handbook of Radiotherapy Physics: Theory and Practice* edited by P Mayles, A Nahum, J C Rosenwald, Copyright 2007. Reproduced with permission of Taylor & Francis Group LLC.

the target with the constricted 90% isodose at a depth, and the proximity of a critical organ at/near the lateral edge of the target volume. This can be a particular problem with small volumes around the nose and cheek, and close to the eyes. In this situation, small irregular shaped fields may be needed. These are produced by cutting out the required field shape from a sheet of lead or low melting point alloy (cleverly called a 'cut-out') from lead sheets or low melting point alloys (LMPAs); clinical data may need to be verified by dose measurements obtained using the patient specific cut-outs.

If the cut-out is too thin, the dose on the surface of the patient, instead of being reduced, may be increased due to the production of forward scattered electrons and bremsstrahlung from the high atomic material on the skin surface (much like X-ray production in a linac target). As a rule of thumb, the minimum thickness of lead required in millimetres is approximately half the mean surface energy of the beam in MeV. For LMPA, typically composed of bismuth, lead, and tin, this should be increased by a factor of 1.2. Generally, this will result in a transmission of less than 5% at lower energies to 10% at 20 MeV.

The ability to join two or more adjacent fields can be useful in a number of clinical situations:

♦ To treat an irregular surface, for example around a chest wall, scalp. This may mean using fields angled towards each other or at right angles; potential overlaps can be mitigated by the use of absorbers at the field edges.

♦ Varying depths across the target volume.

♦ A larger area than a standard applicator, for example skin lymphoma.

However, they do present significant problems due to the shape of the electron isodoses:

♦ A match at the surface edge of abutting fields gives hot spots at a depth.

♦ A match at a depth by leaving a calculated gap at the surface produces a cold spot within the target volume.

♦ Significant differences in hot or cold areas can be produced by small variations in the relative positions of the beams.

These problems can be alleviated by a number of strategies:

♦ Position abutting edges away from any critical area.

♦ Use moving junctions, similar to some photon techniques, for example craniospinal irradiation, to 'smudge out' the overlap area.

♦ Slightly angle beams away from each other to reduce hot spot area.

♦ Use strips of absorbers or energy degraders along the match line.

♦ Doses and dose distributions should be tested experimentally before treatment and perhaps also during treatment in the more complicated circumstances.

♦ Electron arc therapy may be used instead of adjacent fields but the implementation of this type of technique requires significant technical effort.

7.7 **Effects of surface obliquity and inhomogeneities on dose distributions**

7.7.1 **Surface obliquity**

Oblique incidence occurs where there is stand-off from the patient's surface to part of the electron beam (see Figure 7.8), for example treatment of a large area of the chest wall.

If we define an angle α as the angle between the central axis of the beam and the normal to the patient's skin surface, then for

- α less than 20° there is little effect on the depth doses and the isodose curves follow the skin surface;
- α between 20° and 30° the isodose curves still follow the surface but if there is stand-off at edge of the collimated area then the penumbral region is widened;
- α between 40° and 60° the depth dose is reduced and the surface dose is increased; the increase in surface dose may be greater than the loss of fluence due to the accompanying extended SSD producing hot spots;
- α greater than 60° the percentage depth dose no longer has its characteristic shape (more akin to superficial X-rays) the value of the practical range changes and there is a steep increase in the maximum dose.

It is best to angle the field so that the fall off around the collimator edges is equal which reduces the more serious effects of surface obliquity. If this is not possible then the difference could be compensated for by using variable thickness bolus and possibly a higher electron energy.

7.7.2 **Inhomogeneities**

Inhomogeneities influence the dose distribution and depend on:

- Energy and field size of the electron beam,
- Size of the inhomogeneity relative to the field size,
- Its shape and composition.

There are two main effects:

1) Change in absorption and the associated shift in the depth of isodose values; usually most noticeable within a large inhomogeneity and beyond its limit, for example lung beneath a chest wall.

2) Scatter differences between materials; these can be significant for small homogeneities or in the interface region with a large homogeneity.

The scatter effects are complex with a higher proportion of electrons scattered from a high-density region into a low-density region than vice versa. This gives a low dose area within the high-density region or distal to it and conversely a high dose area within a low-density region and beyond it.

The effect is energy dependent, increasing with increasing energy requiring an estimation of the effective electron energy at the depth of the inhomogeneity. A Monte Carlo-based treatment planning system (section 9.14.4) would give the

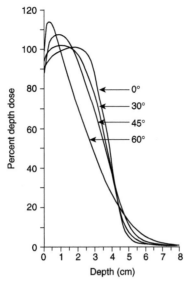

Figure 7.8 The variation in depth dose with variation of angle of incidence along the central axis for 10 MeV electrons: note how the increased angle of incidence beyond 30 degrees leads to a decrease in the depth of the maximum dose, but greater than 60 degrees leads to a large increase in the maximum dose.
Reproduced with permission from Williams and Thwaites, *Radiotherapy Physics in Practice*, 1993, Oxford University Press.

best approximation of these interface effects which can be found in a number of situations:

- Interfaces involving air, lung, and bone,
- Surface irregularities such as shaped bolus, lead cut-outs, nose, ear.

The ear can present significant problems which can be tackled by the use of a tissue equivalent plug, for example wax to circumvent the air/tissue interface.

7.8 **Internal shielding**

Internal shielding is used to spare structures lying below the target volume and is usually encountered in the irradiation of lips, cheek, ear, and eyelids. There is a need to calculate the minimum thickness of shielding material to give the required shielding which is energy dependent. It may be that there will be a restriction on this thickness due to the available space, for example under an eyelid.

Any shielding material will produce backscatter and this will increase the dose at the tissue/shield interface. The excess dose increases with increasing atomic number, Z, of the shielding material and decreasing electron energy and can be significant, with increases over 50% being possible. The use of low Z material, for example dental wax, as a coating mechanism can significantly reduce this excess dose by absorption of the low energy backscattered electrons. Typically, 2 mm of lead is used for shielding with a coating of 8 mm of wax. This may be feasible in the case of the inside of a lip. However, any shielding may be impractical in the case of the inner surface of an eyelid. The use of internal shielding may need a compromise in the prescribed dose.

Chapter 8

Imaging for treatment planning

Frances Lavender and Gemma Whitelaw

8.1 Introduction: what are planning images used for?

Information from planning images is used throughout the patient pathway. It is therefore vital that we understand the limitations and uncertainties associated with these images, and any impact these will have on the accuracy of the dose delivered during treatment. Images need to be fit for purpose, whilst ensuring we keep the dose to the patient as low as reasonably practicable (ALARP) (see Section 14.4).

So what are the main purposes of images used during treatment planning (Figure 8.1)? Images are used to:

1) 'Map' and identify targets and organs at risk (anatomical imaging)

2) Quantify functional parameters (functional imaging)

3) Visualize the change in position of targets or other anatomy with time (four-dimensional (4D) imaging)

4) Measure parameters needed to calculate dose

5) Create 'setup images' which will be used to position the patient at treatment

8.2 The ideal planning dataset

Images are often referred to as a 'dataset'. This is imported into the treatment planning system (TPS) and used to calculate the best treatment plan and dose distribution. So, what would our ideal planning dataset look like? In a perfect world, we want everything in our planning images to exactly match how things will be at treatment. For example, if we are using a 3D CT scan as our planning dataset, we want the patient to be in the same position in the planning dataset as they will be for every fraction of treatment. Additionally, we'd like all of their organs to be in exactly the same position, the same size, and the same density (i.e. the same rectal and bladder filling and no changes in the amount or position of gas in the bowel). It would also be a lot easier if everything within the patient was completely stationary. Some of these factors we can control. Other factors, such as organ motion, we will need to quantify and then use this assessment to inform our choice of planning and treatment techniques. Below are some of the features of an 'ideal' planning dataset.

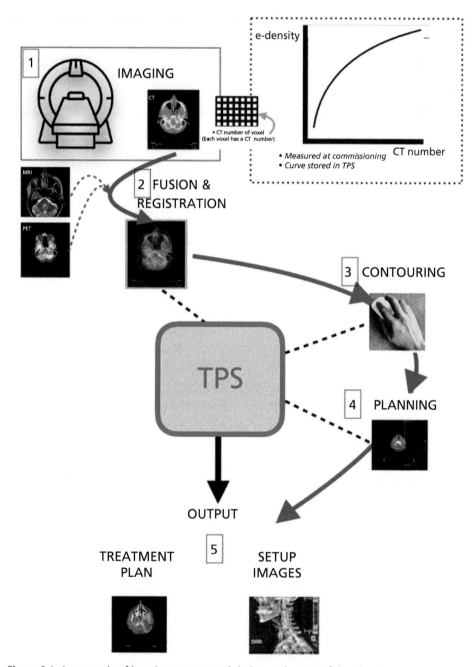

Figure 8.1 An example of how images are used during each stage of the planning process.
Reproduced with permission from RaySearch Laboratories, Stockholm, Sweden

8.2.2 Reproducible patient position

The patient's position at scanning needs to match the patient's position at treatment as much as possible. Diagnostic scanners often have curved couches. Linear accelerators (linacs) have flat couches. Therefore, for planning images we need to put a flat couch-top onto our CT/MRI/PET scanner so that the patient is in a similar position. We also want to scan with the patient in the same immobilization equipment that will be used on the linac during treatment (e.g. shells, footrests, breast boards, 'vacbags', etc.) in order to minimize patient movement and ensure a reproducible setup.

8.2.3 External reference points (patient alignment)

It is useful to have reference points on the imaging dataset that can be used for initial setup of the patient in the treatment room. A common example of this is to use ball bearings and tattoos on the patient's skin. For example, a dedicated Radiotherapy CT scanner room will have in-room lasers that match the lasers in the linac bunker. The patient will be positioned on the CT couch. The radiographers will align the patient to these lasers and mark with pen where the ceiling and wall lasers hit the skin anteriorly and laterally. However, pen marks cannot be seen on a CT scan. Therefore, small metal ball bearings are taped over the pen marks as these will be easily identified on the CT images due to their high density. After the scan, radiographers make the marks permanent by making a small tattoo 'dot' over the pen marks. When the patient has their first treatment session on the linac, they will be positioned on the couch. The couch will then be moved to align the patient's tattoos with the linac room lasers. Further setup moves and imaging will then be performed to fine-tune the patient's position (see Chapter 10).

8.2.4 Position of internal organs

Changes in organ position and shape can be minimized using 'prep' protocols for organ filling (e.g. drinking protocols for bladder filling, enemas for rectal filling). Movement of organs can be determined using 4D imaging techniques. In some cases, fiducial markers may be inserted into an organ. These are usually small high-density markers that can be clearly identified on images and can therefore be used to track organ motion.

8.2.5 Accurate transfer between systems

Images will be exported from the scanner and imported into to the TPS. It is therefore essential that the TPS can 'read' images from all imaging systems without any corruption or loss of data. All imaging systems (e.g. PET, MRI, CT scanners, from all manufacturers) must comply with the Digital Imaging and Communication in Medicine (DICOM) standard to ensure the accurate transfer of data between systems (see Chapter 4).

8.2.6 **Appropriate image quality**

The image quality must be appropriate for the purpose of the images (as listed in section 8.1). For imaging that uses ionizing radiation (e.g. CT and PET) the image quality is intrinsically linked to the dose to the patient. The factors that dictate image quality differ for each imaging modality and are discussed in this chapter.

8.2.7 **Minimize artefacts**

We need the quantitative information in the dataset to be accurate. An artefact is a feature in the image which does not accurately represent the object being imaged. This introduces inaccuracies into the planning dataset. For example, artefacts may change the CT number or standardized uptake values in an image or introduce geometric distortion into the image. Therefore artefacts need to be identified and corrections made to reduce or compensate for these inaccuracies.

8.2.8 **Selection of most useful type of information (anatomical or functional imaging)**

Multiple image datasets are often used to provide different types of information. Anatomical imaging gives us a geometric 'map' of structures. Functional imaging gives an indication of a particular process occurring within the body. Functional information may aid diagnosis, staging, contouring, and choice of treatment regimens. For dose calculation, we will require accurate anatomical information.

8.3 **Computed tomography (CT)**

The most common imaging modality used for radiotherapy planning is computed tomography (CT). Why is this? To answer this we first need to understand how CT images are acquired and reconstructed.

8.3.1 **How do CT scanners work?**

The ring-shaped gantry of the CT scanner contains an X-ray tube and a bank of X-ray detectors. The X-rays emitted from the tube form a 'fan shaped' beam of X-rays across the patient. The tube and detectors rotate around the gantry at speeds of up to 3.3 revolutions per second. There are two main types of CT acquisition:

◆ **Axial** scanning, where the couch is stationary whilst the beam is on. The couch remains in a fixed position whilst the first longitudinal section of the scan is acquired. Once the beam is switched off, the couch moves through the gantry, stops, and then the next longitudinal section of the scan is acquired. The switching on and off of the beam is automated for axial scanning.

◆ **Helical** scanning, where the couch moves through the gantry continuously whilst the beam is on. From the perspective of the patient, the X-ray beam traces a helical path around them.

At each gantry angle, some of the X-ray beam will be attenuated due to photon interactions in the patient, and the remaining X-rays will reach the detectors. What determines how many X-rays will reach the detectors? Let's think back to photon interactions as discussed in Chapter 2.

◆ If the beam travels through regions of high density inside the patient, for example bone or metallic implants, the probability of photon interactions increases compared to that in soft tissue. Consequently, more of the X-ray beam will be attenuated in bone or metal than in soft tissue and fewer photons will reach the detectors.

◆ If the patient is large, the beam must travel a greater distance through tissue (a longer 'path length') than in a smaller patient. As the path length in tissue increases, the probability of a photon interaction occurring also increases and fewer photons will reach the detectors.

Using the number of X-rays detected at each point in the detector bank, the system reconstructs a 3D image using processes such as filtered back projection or iterative reconstruction. The output from this reconstruction is a stack of images, or 'slices'. Each slice consists of a matrix of volume elements (voxels). The voxel size defines the resolution of the image. Each voxel has an associated CT number. The units of CT number are Hounsfield units (HU), defined as:

$$CT\,number\,(HU) = \frac{\mu\,material - \mu\,water}{\mu\,water} \times 1000$$

where μ is the linear attenuation coefficient which is the fraction of the beam that is attenuated per unit thickness of the material. The change in intensity of the beam as it travels through the material is described by the equation,

$$I = Io.e^{-\mu x}$$

where Io is the initial intensity of an X-ray beam and I is the intensity of the X-ray beam after it has travelled a distance x through the material. Some typical CT numbers are shown in Table 8.1. A CT number greater than 0 HU indicates that the material is more attenuating than water. A CT number of less than 0 HU indicates that the material is less attenuating than water.

Table 8.1 Approximate CT numbers for different tissues

Material	CT number (HU)
Bone	300
Muscle	50
Soft tissue	0 to 50
Water	0
Fat	−100
Lung tissue	−200
Air	−1000

In order to visualize this matrix of CT numbers, each CT number is assigned a greyscale value. The range and number of grey levels can be adjusted by 'windowing' the CT image. Windowing will change the appearance of the image, making different tissues brighter or darker, but it does not change the CT number.

8.3.2 Acquisition parameters

Now that we understand the theory behind CT, let's think about the different settings we can use when acquiring our CT scan. These include:

- mA: The X-ray tube current, in units of milliamperes (mA). Refer to section 2.3.5 to remind yourself how mA and kV relate to the number and energy of photons emitted from an X-ray tube. CT scanners use mA modulation to automatically increase and decrease the mA (within a pre-defined range) over regions of the patient which are more or less attenuating.

- mAs: The tube current-time product in units of milliampere-second (mAs) is the product of the tube current with the exposure time per rotation.

- kV: The X-ray tube voltage, in units of kilovolts (kV). Dual-energy CT is described in section 8.3.5.

- Slice thickness and acquired resolution: The detector array in a CT scanner consists of many small detector elements. For example, a 64-slice CT scanner may have an array consisting of 64 rows of detector elements, each of length 0.5 mm in the direction of the long-axis of the couch. The smallest acquisition slice thickness achievable on such a scanner would usually be 0.5 mm. This would give a resolution along the long-axis of the patient of 0.5 mm. Selecting the smallest acquisition slice thickness may however lead to a long scan time and a larger dose to the patient than is necessary. If a resolution of 0.5 mm is not required for the planning dataset, detector rows can be grouped together at acquisition to increase the slice thickness, thereby minimizing both the dose to the patient and the scan time.

8.3.3 Reconstruction parameters

After the scan has been acquired, post-processing techniques can be used to alter the properties of the image.

- Filters, kernels: Image-processing filters or kernels can be applied to change how the image appears. For example, these can make the image look 'smoother' or less noisy, alter the contrast, or make edges look sharper.

- Reconstructed resolution: The minimum resolution in the longitudinal axis is limited by the size of the detector element. However, after the scan, the operator can re-reconstruct the dataset into larger slice thicknesses by combining the data from groups of detector elements.

- Metal artefact reduction: Another common algorithm applied to CT scans is metal artefact reduction. If metal is present in the patient (e.g. dental fillings, implants), the beam is highly attenuated. This can result in a 'streak' artefact (see Figure 10.3). Algorithms can reduce these artefacts by estimating what the CT number might be if no metal was present and changing the CT number in the affected voxels.

Operators involved in planning must be aware that reconstruction parameters can change the CT number or geometric accuracy in an image. These effects of this will be measured by physicists during commissioning of the CT scanner.

8.3.4 Understanding imaging statistics and dose in CT

Let's look at how image quality is related to dose. What happens if we increase the mAs of a CT protocol?

Increasing the mAs → increases the current through the X-ray tube cathode → more electrons are emitted from the cathode → more photons are emitted at the anode → more photons will therefore reach the detectors. This results in a better image as shown in Figure 8.2. However, more photons emitted at the anode also means that more photons will be incident on the patient and therefore more photons will be attenuated in tissue, resulting in an increased dose to the patient.

8.3.5 Dual-energy CT

Dual-energy CT scanners use X-ray beams of two different energies (e.g. 80 and 140 kV) to create the CT dataset. By using a variety of reconstruction techniques, the dual-energy dataset can give improved contrast, a reduction in artefacts, or information about the chemical composition of materials.

8.3.6 CT calibration curve in the TPS

What information is required by the treatment planning system to enable it to calculate dose? In order to calculate the probability of photon interactions in tissue, the TPS needs to know the electron or mass density of different tissues. However, a CT scan does not directly contain this information. Therefore, we need to tell the TPS how to 'convert' the CT number into either electron density (number of electrons per unit volume) or mass density. This is done by setting up a calibration curve that defines the relationship between CT number and electron or mass density for that specific CT scanner. When a new CT scanner is commissioned, physicists will measure this calibration curve using a phantom that contains inserts of different densities (Figure 8.3).

(a)   (b)

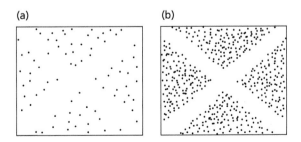

- Imaging for Treatment Planning
- Understanding imaging statistics and dose in CT

Figure 8.2 Images created with a large number of photons (b) appear less 'noisy' than images created with fewer photons (a), but will result in a higher dose to the patient.

(a)   (b)

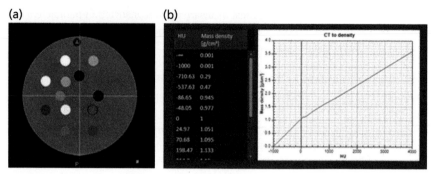

Figure 8.3 A phantom containing inserts of different materials used to measure the CT number for a range of materials (a). The resulting CT number (HU) to mass density (g/cm³) calibration curve that is put into the TPS (b).
Reproduced with permission from RaySearch Laboratories, Stockholm, Sweden

The electron and mass densities of the inserts are provided by the manufacturer. The physicist will scan the phantom and measure the CT number of each insert. The CT number is then plotted against the electron density or mass density. This calibration curve is then input into the TPS. The planning system will use this calibration curve when calculating dose for every patient that is scanned on that specific CT scanner.

The calibration curve will be dependent on the energy of the X-ray beam. Consequently, most centres use a single kV setting for all their radiotherapy planning scan CT protocols so that the same calibration curve can be used for all images.

8.4 IR(ME)R and concomitant exposures in RT

Concomitant exposures are defined under Ionising Radiation (Medical Exposure) Regulations (IR(ME)R) (Section 14.7.2) as all exposures within a course of radiotherapy other than treatment exposures. These will therefore include pre-treatment images from ionising modalities such as CT or PET, and on-treatment setup and verification images. IR(ME)R states that practitioners and operators must ensure that doses arising from concomitant exposures are kept ALARP consistent with the intended purpose. CT protocols must therefore be optimised, so that they give the required image quality whilst minimising the dose to the patient. Acquisition and reconstruction parameters will be tested by Physics when the CT scanner is commissioned. The optimal parameters for each scan type will be stored as a list of protocols on the scanner.

EXAMPLE: OPTIMIZING CT PROTOCOLS

Your department has bought a new CT scanner for radiotherapy. You are asked to work with a physicist and radiographer to set up the scanning protocols. All the CT protocols will use 120 kV. What other parameters might you choose for the following scan types: (a) orbits, (b) pelvis, (c) head and neck?

Answer: (a) use a thin slice thickness to achieve good resolution over small regions of anatomy such as orbits, lenses, optic nerves, (b) wide part of the body containing large volume of bones; therefore use high enough mAs to achieve the necessary image quality, but keep ALARP to minimize dose to the patient, (c) dental fillings may result in steaking artefacts in the image; use a metal artefact algorithm to reduce this.

8.5 Other types of images commonly used in RT planning

8.5.1 Ultrasound

Ultrasound (US) is a non-ionizing imaging modality that utilizes sound waves at frequencies above that of human hearing (> 20 kHz).

High-frequency sound waves are created in a piezoelectric crystal in a transducer; these sound waves advance into the tissue being scanned by way of a water-based gel. The sound waves reflect at boundaries of tissue with different acoustic impedance. These echoed waves are detected, again by the piezoelectric crystal, and are translated into an electrical signal from which an image may be formed. Images are created by interrogating the length of time it takes for each echo to be detected by the transducer; tissue boundaries at greater depth cause a longer time difference between generation and detection of the ultrasound. The returned ultrasound intensity is also used.

A range of transducers are available, selected for the anatomical area of interest and focus required. Curvilinear transducers are generally used for abdominal imaging, whereas smaller, wider field of view transducers are more suitable for transvaginal and transrectal imaging. Whilst most imaging is in two dimensions representing the acoustic impedance across one plane of tissue; ultrasound can be used for forming both 3D and 4D images. By means of the Doppler Effect, ultrasound may also be used to monitor and measure moving objects within the body, this is put into practice in blood flow imaging.

In the Radiotherapy department transabdominal ultrasound is employed for bladder volume measurements prior to external beam treatment. Good bladder preparation and consistency in volume are important in the accurate delivery of radiation. Ultrasound is also routinely used to locate the correct placement of brachytherapy applicators, for example ensuring the correct siting of a vaginal cylinder prior to high dose rate radiotherapy.

Ultrasound is widely used in low dose rate prostate brachytherapy. A transrectal probe, with perpendicular piezoelectric arrays, is used to image the patient volumetrically prior to planning, in a similar way that a CT volume is used for external beam planning. The ultrasound is then utilized to guide the surgeon and physicist in the real-time placement of the radioactive sources.

A robust quality assurance regime should be employed when using ultrasound, such as that outlined in available professional guidance, particularly regarding image resolution, signal to noise ratio and distance and volume measurements.

8.5.2 PET

Positron emission tomography (PET) is a type of functional imaging which uses positron-emitting radiopharmaceuticals.

Some radioisotopes have nuclei that contain more protons than neutrons. This makes the nucleus unstable. To transform into a more stable state the radioisotope may decay via positron emission (see section 1.5.4), where a proton changes to a neutron and a positron is emitted. A positron is an anti-matter electron. It has the same mass as an electron but a charge of +1. If a positron encounters an electron, it may interact via an 'annihilation event' where the positron and electron transfer their energy to two 511 keV photons.

By attaching a radioisotope to a substance that is involved in a specific physiological process, we can see not only where this process occurs but also information about the timescales involved with this process. For example, the radioisotope fluorine-18 (^{18}F) can be attached to a glucose analogue such as fluorodeoxyglucose (FDG) to create the radiopharmaceutical ^{18}F-FDG. This can be injected into the bloodstream and will then be absorbed by tissues. Positrons will annihilate with electrons in the tissue and some of the resulting 511 keV photons will escape the body and be detected by a ring of detectors around the patient. By using a glucose analogue, the image will highlight regions of high metabolic activity. Another commonly used radiopharmaceutical is carbon-11 choline (^{11}C-choline) which will highlight regions of metabolic activity of phospholipids in the cell membrane. The standardized uptake value (SUV) gives an indication of tracer uptake in a region, whilst considering parameters such as injected dose and patient weight.

PET scanners usually have an in-built CT scanner (PET-CT scanners). This allows PET and CT images to be taken consecutively, without the patient having to move between scans. The CT data provide anatomical information and is also used to perform corrections on the PET data such as attenuation correction.

8.5.3 MRI

Magnetic resonance imaging (MRI) uses magnetic fields and radiofrequency (RF) pulses to manipulate the spin of protons and detect the RF energy emitted as protons return to their original state.

MRI utilizes a quantum mechanical property of particles called 'spin'. In simplified terms, we can consider protons to act like small bar magnets. The MRI scanner produces a strong magnetic field. Protons in tissue tend to align in a magnetic field. The scanner delivers RF pulses which 'excite' the protons. As the protons 'relax' back into their original energy state, RF energy is emitted, detected by a receiver, and reconstructed to create the MR image.

The human body has a high composition of water and hence hydrogen molecules. The nucleus of a hydrogen molecule is a single proton. Due to both the properties of hydrogen nuclei and its abundance in the body, the signal from hydrogen is typically used to produce MR images. By using different sequences of fields and RF pulses, different tissues or processes can be highlighted as shown in Figure 8.4.

(a)   (b)   (c)

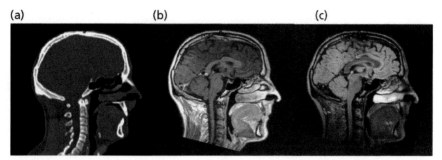

Figure 8.4 Three images acquired prior to planning for external beam radiotherapy to the brain. Planning CT (a), a T1 sequence MRI (b), a T2 FLAIR sequence MRI (c).
Reproduced with permission from RaySearch Laboratories, Stockholm, Sweden

8.5.3.1 Can MR images be used to calculate dose?

MR images are based on the properties of protons. They do not directly tell us the electron density of tissues, which is what we need for the TPS to calculate dose. However, if we can identify the type of tissue in each MRI voxel, we can apply CT numbers to each voxel to create a 'pseudo-CT' image. This can then be used with an appropriate calibration curve to estimate dose.

8.5.4 **4D imaging**

Four-dimensional (4D) imaging incorporates the dimension of time when reconstructing 3D (volumetric) data. This allows us to capture movement that occurred during the scan.

Let's consider a 4D CT lung scan. We need to know which part of the respiration cycle corresponds to each section of the CT scan. Therefore, the respiration cycle will be recorded for the duration of the CT scan. There are different ways to measure this. For example: a plastic block with infrared reflectors can be placed on the patient's skin and infrared cameras used to detect motion of the block; movement of a specified structure within the body (e.g. part of a rib) can act as a surrogate, or the volume of air breathed into a mouthpiece can be measured. To have images that show the position of the tumour at different points in the respiratory cycle, the trace is divided into a number of sections or 'bins' (Figure 8.5). For each bin, image data are summed from every couch position and reconstructed. This will give an image of the lung that correlates to a specific amplitude or phase range of the respiratory cycle. By playing these sets of images in order, a movie-like 'cine image' is created, which shows motion over the whole respiratory cycle.

So if 4D CT allows us to visualise organ movement, why don't we use 4D CT for all of our planning images? If we have 10 bins, we have effectively created 10 separate 3D CT datasets. To achieve appropriate image quality for this the acquisition time is longer and the total dose to the patient is higher compared to a 3D CT scan.

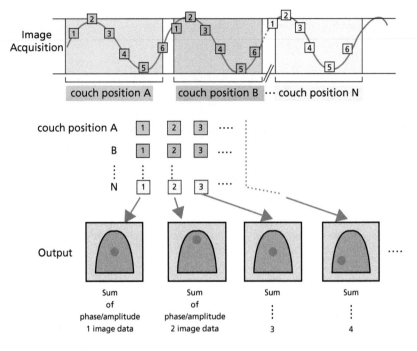

- Imaging for Treatment Planning
- 4D imaging

Figure 8.5 A simplified diagram of how 4DCT works. The patient's respiratory cycle is recorded throughout the CT scan (green sinusoidal line). Imaging data is divided into 'bins' (6 bins for this simplified example. Clinically data would be divided into at least 10bins). Data for each time bin is summed over all couch positions.

EXAMPLE: 4D CT

A colleague suggests that a 4D CT scan is requested for two patients to be used for radiotherapy planning of external beam treatment on a linac. If you are the practitioner, what is your role under IR(ME)R and is a 4D CT scan appropriate for each patient?

(A) PATIENT 1: Radiotherapy to a small lesion in the apex of the left lung. The 4D CT is requested to assess motion of the tumour.

(B) PATIENT 2: Radiotherapy to the prostate and nodes. The 4D CT is requested to assess motion of bowel adjacent to the nodal PTV.

Answers: The practitioner is responsible for justifying the radiation exposure. For patient 1 a 4D CT may be justified as it will provide information about how the tumour moves during respiration. This can lead to a more targeted radiotherapy treatment. For patient 2, the 4D scan will show the position of the bowel at the time of scanning. However, it is unlikely that the bowel will be in the same position during each treatment fraction. The higher dose from a 4D CT scan would not be justified for this case as no additional information is gained from the 4D CT that could not be ascertained from a lower dose 3D CT scan.

8.5.5 What type of imaging is best?

The most appropriate imaging modality will depend on its purpose. Table 8.2 summarises the main features of four types of images.

Table 8.2 A summary of the main features of four types of imaging modality commonly used in radiotherapy planning

	CT	MRI	PET	U/S
Features	◆ Photons are emitted from an X-ray tube and undergo photon interactions in tissue. ◆ CT number quantifies attenuation of photons. ◆ A calibration curve is used to convert CT number (HU) to electron density. ◆ The TPS uses electron density to calculate dose.	◆ Protons act like small magnets and tend to align with external magnetic fields. ◆ Radiofrequency pulses 'excite' the protons. ◆ As the protons 'relax' back into their original state they emit RF energy which is detected by receivers.	◆ A positron-emitting radiopharmaceutical is administered. ◆ Positrons interact with electrons in tissue, transferring their energy to two 511 keV photons. ◆ Photons escape from the body and are detected.	◆ High-frequency soundwaves are transmitted from a transducer to tissue. ◆ At boundaries between materials of different densities, some of the soundwaves are reflected and then detected by the ultrasound probe.
Advantages	✓ Excellent anatomical information, not subject to significant geometric distortion ✓ Short acquisition times ✓ Excellent resolution	✓ Different MRI sequences can provide anatomical and functional information ✓ Excellent soft tissue contrast ✓ No radiation dose	✓ Functional information from PET is usually inherently registered to anatomical information from CT (PET-CT) ✓ High sensitivity	✓ Real-time functional and anatomical information (adaptive planning) ✓ US probe can be positioned close to treatment area (e.g. transrectal for prostate brachytherapy) ✓ Inexpensive ✓ No radiation dose
Disadvantages	✗ Radiation dose ✗ Poor soft tissue contrast ✗ Artefacts from high density materials (e.g. metal)	✗ Geometric distortion ✗ Acquisition times can be long for high resolution images ✗ Ferromagnetic materials (e.g. some implants) cannot be brought near the MRI scanner.	✗ Radiation dose ✗ Limited resolution ✗ Acquisition times can be long	✗ Imaging large volumes introduces geometric distortion

8.6 **Registration/fusion**

If multiple imaging datasets are imported into the TPS, these need to be 'aligned' to each other. This process is called image registration or fusion. For example, a patient may have had a CT planning scan (let's call this the primary image) and multiple MRI scans of the brain using different MRI sequences (let's call these secondary images) on the same day. So why don't these images automatically align with each other when imported into the TPS? First, the CT scan and the MRI scanners have different co-ordinate systems, so the 'centre' of the CT scan is not the same as the 'centre' of the MR image. Secondly, even though we will try to match the setup of the patient in the two scanners as closely as possible (by using a flat couch, the same immobilization devices, or the same bladder/rectum filling protocols for pelvis patients), there will always be setup differences. Finally, the scan time for multiple MRI sequences can take from a few minutes up to half an hour. The patient will not remain completely stationary for this time and internal organs definitely will not! So MR images from different acquisition sequences may require registration with each other.

So, upon opening the images in the TPS, the dosimetrist or physicist will register the secondary images to the primary image using selected anatomical landmarks such as bones, soft tissue, external contours, or fiducials. It is often not possible to align all parts of the images exactly, so it is important to consider which part of the scan is the most appropriate part to align. Usually registration will be optimised on the region around the target, as this is where the secondary image datasets will be used to contour the gross tumour volume (GTV) and clinical target volume (CTV). It is essential that registration is accurate, as any errors in registration will decrease the targeting accuracy of the radiotherapy treatment. Consequently, clinicians should always check the registration before contouring.

8.6.1 **Rigid and deformable registration**

The above section describes rigid registration. This means that each image may be translated, rotated, magnified, or shrunk, but not distorted. Every voxel in an image is translated, magnified, or shrunk by the same amount, or rotated about the same point of rotation. This will provide a good match between images if there are no anatomical changes between the two image sets. (See Figures 8.6a-c).

In non-rigid, or 'deformable' registration, the grid of voxels can be 'warped', that is different voxels undergo different transformations. This is especially useful when there are changes such as shrinkage of the tumour, weight loss, or changes in organ shape. (See Figures 8.6d-e).

8.7 **Contouring**

Now that we have a beautifully registered set of images, the clinician will contour the target structures and organs at risk. The exposure parameters of the scans will have been optimised at scanning to provide the appropriate image quality for contouring

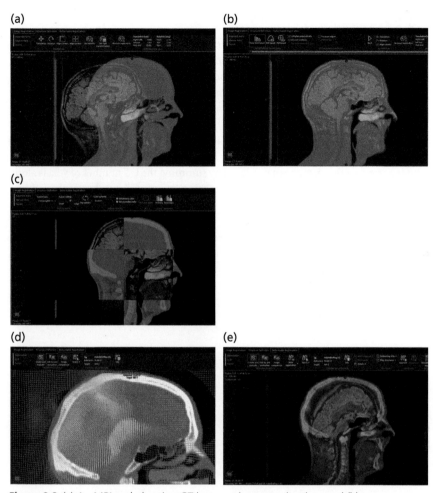

Figure 8.6 (a) An MRI and planning CT image prior to regsitration, and (b) once registered. Toolbars above the image show the tools available for manual (a) or automatic regsitration (b) in this software.
(c) A variety of display settings, such as this 'checkers' view, may be used by the operator to check the accuracy or the registration.
(d) Deformable registration. A vector display illustrating how the image mesh is 'warped', and (e) the resulting deformed image (right). For this example the MRI has been deliberately deformed in a non-clinicial way to illustrate the effect of large vectors.
Reproduced with permission from RaySearch Laboratories, Stockholm, Sweden

whist keeping the concomitant dose to the patient ALARP. Whilst contouring, the clinician needs to be aware of which image set will be used for dose calculation, and the magnitude of uncertainties due to registration. Once contouring is complete, the next stage is planning (see Chapter 9).

8.8 **Setup images**

So the patient arrives for fraction 1 and lies on the linac couch in the treatment room. How do we know if the patient is in the same position as they were for their planning CT? After initial alignment to tattoos, and moves from the tattoos to the planning isocentre, imaging will usually be performed. These are often called 'on-set' images. This is discussed in section 10.1. At the planning stage, we will create setup images that can be compared to the on-set images.

A common type of setup image is a digitally reconstructed radiograph (DRR). These are 2D images, created from the planning CT dataset. Therefore they can look like a planar X-ray, but they have been produced by summing the CT number of voxels along a projection through the CT dataset. By choosing to sum CT numbers only within a selected range (e.g. those associated with bone), the DRR can be manipulated to look like a planar X-ray (e.g. to clearly see bones in the DRR). Similarly, different ranges can be selected to maximise the contrast between tissues of different densities such as air/ lung and soft tissue (e.g. to see the patient surface and chest wall for breast treatments) or to see high density objects such as fiducials (e.g. for prostate treatments). An example of a DRR is shown in Figure 10.1.

Chapter 9

External beam treatment planning

Christopher Dean, Niall MacDougall, and Andrew Morgan

9.1 What do we need for treatment planning?

Treatment planning is the process of taking data that pertain to the patient, as described in Chapter 8, along with the data that pertain to the linear accelerator (linac) treatment beam to create a set of instructions and parameters that allow us to deliver a known dose to a region inside a patient. However, this one term covers a very wide range of dosimetric complexity.

The simplest treatment plan we can imagine is one of a single field at normal incidence to a patient surface. The simplicity of this kind of plan indicates it is likely to be of palliative intent and so might not warrant the use of a treatment planning system (TPS) in order to define the treatment parameters.

At the other end of the spectrum is full online-adaptive treatment planning using modulated beam delivery (see section 9.10) to deliver a radical dose based on the anatomical positions of target(s) and/or organ(s) at risk and their relationship on the day of treatment. This type of radiotherapy would certainly warrant the use of (at least one) TPS to ensure that the intended dose is delivered to the patient as accurately as possible.

While the topics of patient positioning, immobilization, imaging for determination of target position, organ motion, and the building of a virtual electronic model of the patient for treatment planning are discussed in detail in Chapter 8, this chapter concentrates on rationale for various methods of treatment planning, the steps involved, and dose calculations.

9.2 Beam parameters required for treatment planning

We saw in Chapter 6 how the configurable beam parameters affect the radiation dose characteristics of the radiation beam when measured in a water bath (phantom). As a reminder, the dominant characteristics of the beam that we use in treatment planning are as follows.

9.2.1 Central axis depth dose

This factor tells us how dose varies along the central axis as a function of distance from the surface. It is defined as percentage depth dose (PDD) if we have a fixed source-to-surface distance (SSD), or tissue maximum ratio (TMR) if we are considering the fixed source-to-axis distance (SAD) for isocentric treatments.

- Fixed SSD setting: each incremental increase in depth (d) from the surface of the patient to the point of interest is both deeper (more attenuating material above it) *and* further from the source of radiation (therefore it has an inverse square law element—section 2.7);
- Fixed SAD (isocentric) setting: each incremental change in depth only means more attenuating material above it as the distance between the source of radiation and the point of interest remains constant (no inverse square law changes). For this reason, the TMR curve is less steep beyond the depth of maximum dose, d_{max}, than the equivalent PDD for the same beam energy (Figure 9.1).

Depth dose also varies with beam energy, collimated field size, inhomogeneity, and due to the presence or absence of a wedge or beam flattening filter in the field.

9.2.2 **Output factor**

This factor tells us how dose varies at a fixed point on the central axis at d_{max} as the field size is varied, keeping everything else fixed (see Figure 6.11).

It is a non-linear function that has two components, namely collimator scatter factor and phantom scatter factor. The most dramatic effects are seen at the smaller end of the field size range where the distance between the collimated field edge and the central axis approaches the lateral distance an electron is likely to travel for that beam energy.

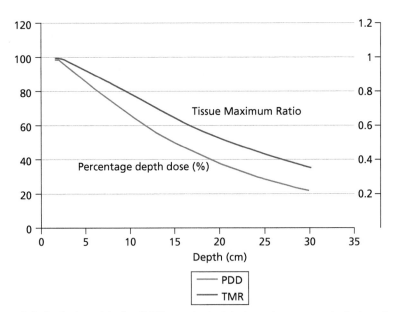

Figure 9.1 depth dose data for 6MV beam (only data from dmax onwards displayed). Note that dmax is identical for both curves.

The dose per machine output starts to drop rapidly on the central axis below this limit as lateral electronic equilibrium starts to break down.

Output factor also varies with beam energy, and whether there is a wedge in the field.

9.2.3 Beam profile

This factor tells us how dose varies across a line perpendicular to the beam central axis, usually along the beam major axes (see Figure 6.7). Beam profiles vary with beam energy, depth, collimated field size, and whether there is a wedge in the field.

At the time the linac and/or the TPS is being commissioned, all these data are collected by direct measurement in water by the radiotherapy physicist. After adequate data checks, these basic measured data are then input in to the TPS. This is used by the TPS to generate the 'beam model'. There are various means of using these data to create the beam model depending on the TPS. This beam model is then used alongside the patient image data to calculate (model) the absorbed dose inside the patient. The various levels of calculation sophistication used to calculate dose in the patient are explained in more detail in section 9.14. Dose calculation models are usually referred to as algorithms.

As well as the measured data going in to the TPS, it is standard practice to have a copy of (at least) depth dose data and output factor data represented in tabular/graphical form and/or in independent calculation software. The reason for this is to facilitate manual calculations to calculate the linac settings required to deliver the simpler radiotherapy treatments. There is more on manual calculations in section 9.7.

9.3 Isodose distributions for simple field arrangements

The earliest TPSs directly used the simple combination of depth dose information (a one-dimensional function) and profile information (a one-dimensional function) to model and display dose distributions in a patient in two dimensions (2D). Although TPSs are much more sophisticated these days in their generation of absorbed dose, this combination of two sets of 1D data is illustrative of how isodoses arise. Isodose lines connect points that receive equal absorbed dose within the patient in the same way that contour lines on a map connect points of equal height above sea level. In three dimensions (2D profile + 1D depth dose), dose is displayed as an isodose surface.

By understanding the features 1D depth dose and 1D profiles from simple beam arrangements, the formulation of 2D isodose distributions from simple beam arrangements can be recognized quite readily and familiarity with these simple cases is useful in understanding clinical dose distributions.

9.3.1 The single field arrangement

Figure 9.2 shows the isodose distribution from a single 6 MV photon beam normally incident on a water phantom with 100 cm SSD. The distribution is normalized to 100% (red) at d_{max} on the central axis.

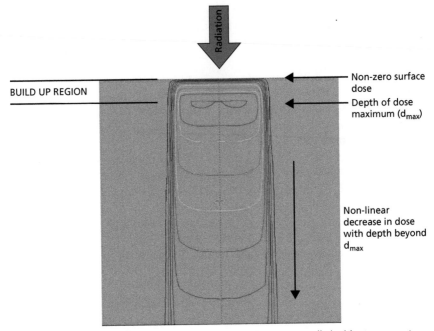

Figure 9.2 Isodose distribution from a 6MV photon beam normally incident on a water phantom at 100cm FSD (100% red, 95% purple, 90% yellow then in 10% increments down to 10% dose).

Features of note:

1) Non-zero dose at the patient surface arising from low energy scattered radiation from the treatment head, backscatter from the superficial parts of the patient and in-air ionization of electrons in the air between the treatment head and the patient surface;

2) Very closely spaced isodose lines from the surface to d_{max} indicating rapidly increasing dose in the build-up region;

3) An increased spacing between the 10% dose increments beyond d_{max} indicating a non-linear depth dose curve with the gradient becoming increasingly shallow at deeper depths;

4) The widening of the penumbrae with depth indicating a mixture of the effect of increased geometric penumbrae further from the beam collimation and the increased contribution of low energy scattered dose at depth;

5) Increased rounding of the isodoses with depth indicating effect of differential beam hardening across the beam due to the shape of the flattening filter (see section 11.3.2.2) Photons nearer the central axis are on average higher energy because they have passed through more material in the high-density flattening filter, similar to the effect discussed for wedges in section 6.5.2.3. The last two effects act to increase the field size required to cover a target volume by a specified isodose level as the depth of the target within the patient increases.

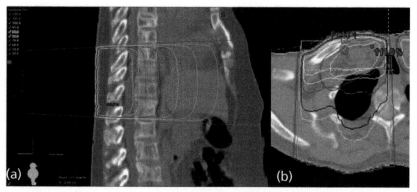

Figure 9.3 Clinical examples of single field arrangements. (a) sagittal projection of treatment for MSCC, 20Gy in 5 fractions is prescribed to the 100% isodose (cyan). The anterior vertebral body receives a heterogeneous dose of between just less than 100% posteriorly and just greater than 80% anteriorly. The spinal cord receives a maximum dose of less than 110% of prescribed dose (salmon) which is less than tolerance for neurological sequelae. (b) Axial projection of treatment for the right supraclavicular fossa, prescription dose 40Gy in 15 fractions with the radiotherapy target (red) largely covered with the 90% isodose (blue). Note the reduced point dose maximum compared with the MSCC example because of the reduce depth to the distal edge of the target (in this case the posterior edge of the fossa).

This type of configuration is used to treat conditions such as metastatic spinal cord compression (MSCC) as it can be planned, checked, and delivered very rapidly without a TPS. However, it suffers from high levels of dose heterogeneity though the target in the beam traversal direction (Figure 9.3). The typical gradient of a 6 MV PDD beyond max is ~4–5%/cm and so to treat a vertebral metastatic deposit of 4 cm thickness, there would exist a 16–20% dose heterogeneity throughout the target. This might be acceptable for this clinical indication where the dose homogeneity is less critical and the spinal cord dose tolerance is still respected.

However for deeper targets where, in order to achieve the desired dose at the tumour, the superficial doses must be much higher to counteract the exponentially decreasing depth dose curve, the simple nature of this arrangement can lead to unacceptably high superficial doses and becomes no longer sufficient.

9.3.2 The parallel opposed pair arrangement

The next level of sophistication is the parallel opposed pair (POP). Figure 9.4 depicts this scenario, where the percentage depth dose from one beam partially counteracts the depth dose from the other resulting in a much more homogeneous dose across the width of the patient. There remains some heterogeneity that is dependent on the beam energy and the width of the patient. The maximum dose in the patient exists at the depths of d_{max}. Beam parameters are set typically such that the dose in the centre of the patient (termed mid-separation) is equal to 100% of the prescription dose by correct choice of monitor units (see section 9.7.4) and that the difference between

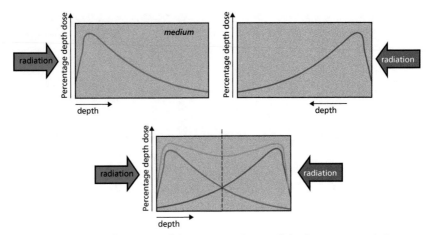

Figure 9.4 Schematic illustration of the concept of a parallel pair arrangement. Green line is the direct summation of the red and blue depth dose lines. Dotted line illustrates position of mid-separation.

the mid-separation dose and the maximum dose is minimized (by choice of beam energy).

Example isodosimetry can be seen in Figure 9.5 where the phantom width is 16 cm and the energy is 6 MV. The hot spot is less than 105% and 95% dose coverage is maintained at mid-separation.

Although this configuration has the benefit over a single field of reducing dose heterogeneity across the target, note that the irradiated volume is significantly larger, and more of the patient receives dose that is greater than prescription dose with the highest doses typically being in areas more superficial than the deep-seated tumour itself.

The POP fields do not have to be equally weighted (or even the same beam energy). These parameters can be modified to shift the prescription dose towards one surface or another (Figure 9.5b). Note how, compared with Figure 9.5b, this uneven distribution allows for more homogeneous dose over a target residing nearer the top of the image and the dose-sparing of the highest doses nearer the bottom of the image, this is at the expense of a significantly larger volume high dose near the top of the image.

This configuration can be seen used to treat deep-seated tumours with palliative intent, such as lung or pelvic cancers (example in Figure 9.6). In all cases the choice of beam energy and weighting will determine the distribution of dose inside the patient and over the tumour volume.

9.3.3 The four field 'brick' configuration

This arrangement is as a result of combining two POPs at right-angles. The high dose area becomes a square or rectangle defined by the region where all four fields overlap. An example for the case of equally sized and weighted fields is shown in Figure 9.7.

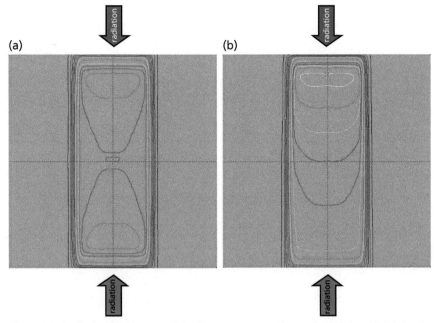

Figure 9.5 isodosimetry from parallel pair arrangement. (a) equally weighted fields (1:1); (b) unequally weighted fields (2:1 in favour of the blue beam). The dose distributions are both designed such that 100% dose (red) is defined at mid-separation, isodoses are at 10% intervals with the addition of the 95% (blue) and 103% (orange), 105% (yellow), 110% (orange) and 115% (white).

Note how there is a large reduction in the superficial (entrance) doses compared with the parallel opposed pair arrangement (Figure 9.6) and also the large reduction in patient volume irradiated to the highest doses. However these two benefits are at the expense of an increased volume of patient being irradiated to the lower levels (40% isodose in dark blue).

Entrance dose (relative to the dose at isocentre (see section 11.3.5)) increases with the depth of the isocentre and where entrance doses become intolerably high the beam energy might be modified upwards to counteract the depth dose curve or the weighting of the fields might be modified.

As the number of fields is increased further (at the extreme end being arc treatments where the patient is irradiated from all gantry approaches) this effect is amplified, that is the volume of patient irradiated to the highest doses reduces as the plan becomes increasingly more conformal to the radiotherapy target but the volume of patient exposed to lower doses (sometimes called the low dose bath) increases.

9.3.4 The effect of wedging

Wedges (discussed in section 6.5) are filters in the head of the linac that modify the field profile in one dimension (Figure 9.8). This effect 'tilts' isodose curves within a field so that they no longer lie perpendicular to the beam central axis.

(a) (b)

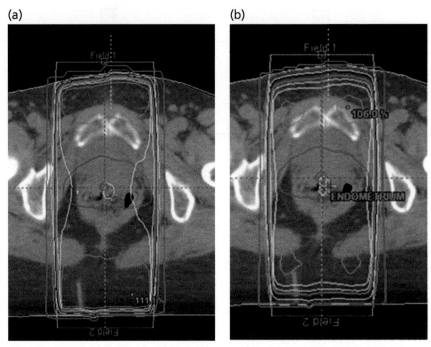

Figure 9.6 Clinical example of a simple parallel opposed pair arrangement used in the palliation of pelvic disease. Both arrangements are equally weighted and both are planned such that the dose at mid separation is 100% of prescription dose (cyan). (a) 6MV fields; B 15MV fields. Note how in (b) the isodoses are more widely spaced in the build-up regions, the dose maxima are lower, and the central target (red contour) is better covered laterally.

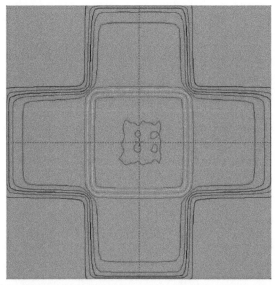

Figure 9.7 Isodose distribution resulting from a four field brick field arrangement, normalized to 100% (red).

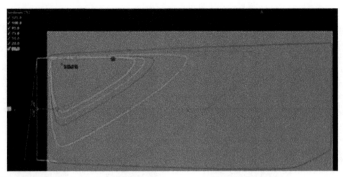

Figure 9.8 The effect of wedges on isodoses.

The angle through which the isodose curves are tilted is known as the wedge angle and there is typically a range through which this is possible (from 10 degrees to 60 degrees) and are used in treatment planning to counteract:

◆ **Beam overlap**, where there is significant dose heterogeneity over the irradiated volume. This is seen in the three-field arrangement (Figure 9.9) for example in anal cancer or the wedged pair arrangement in the treatment of parotid tumours;

◆ **Entrance obliquity**, where the central axis of the beam is not normal to the surface of the patient. This usually means that there is a variation in distance between the surface and the plane of interest across at least one of the beam major axes. An example of this is in the tangential arrangement for breast cancer where the superficial edge has a much shorter path length than the deeper edge of the field. The wedge(s) in this case would be thick end anterior (superficial) as indicated in Figure 9.10 b;

◆ **Internal anatomical variation in radiological path length**. An example of this is in the treatment of the lung and mediastinum where the mid-sagittal radiological path length (section 9.5) can be significantly larger than the parasagittal equivalent. The wedge in this case would be thick end lateral.

(a)   (b)

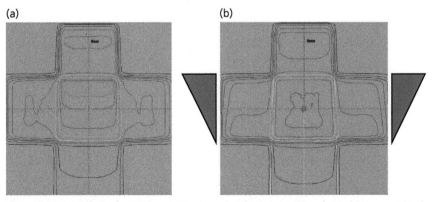

Figure 9.9 The effect of wedging. (a) isodose distribution resulting from three unwedged fields at right angles; (b) modification by using 45 degree wedges on the left and right lateral fields as indicated.

(a) (b)

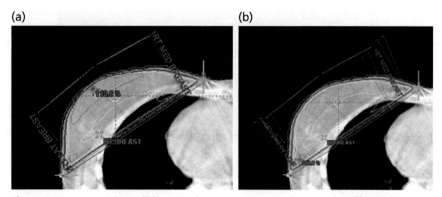

Figure 9.10 Tangential parallel opposed pair arrangement showing the effects of the wedge. (a) no wedges used and a large heterogeneity seen (105% isodose orange); (b) applied wedges reducing the heterogeneity markedly.

9.4 The difference between fixed SSD (source-to-surface) and isocentric plans

The very simplest treatment setup is when we use a single field. Sets of PDD data are collected when the treatment machine is commissioned (see section 11.8.3). PDD curves are dependent on SSD (see section 6.3.3). Linacs are built with the source to isocentre distance set at 100 cm. Therefore, for ease and simplicity, for single field treatments, the SSD is set so the skin is at the isocentre (100 cm from the source). We term this 100 cm fixed SSD treatment.

However, when a second field is added the situation becomes more complicated. We already know that percentage depth dose is a function of SSD because the inverse-square law is at play in PDD and this changes with distance from the source (section 6.3.3). We would now need *different* PDD data for field 2 since the SSD is no longer at 100 cm for this second field. Indeed, we would need this for every field where the SSD was not 100 cm. Before the widespread use of TPSs, combining multiple treatment fields each with a different SSD in order to produce a combined dose distribution was not a practical possibility.

To overcome this (in the example of a POP), one option is to treat field 1 and then reset the patient such that field 2 SSD was also 100 cm, thus removing the need for a large amount of PDD data for all potential SSD values. Calculation of the total dose fields is now straightforward as the fixed SSD isodose distributions or PDDs are simply added together in a ratio defined by the field weighting. However, in terms of delivery this remains time consuming as the patient position would have to be changed between fields for the correct setup. Risk of error is raised from this additional repositioning of the patient. This would also reduce patient throughput as resetting the patient between fields takes time.

A better option, rather than fixing the SSD, would be to fix the source-to-axis distance (SAD), putting the centre of the tumour at the linac isocentre (axis). This is termed *isocentric* (same centre) treatment and the linac can be moved around the patient from outside the treatment room with the minimum of intervention.

This means that for a typical, non-cylindrical, patient the SSD can be different for each treatment field; however, because the distance between the source and measurement point (isocentre) is fixed, we have removed the effect of the inverse square law because this is identical for all fields. Now the dose is only a function of the TMR (section 6.6.3.5), that is amount of attenuation resulting from overlaying material between the patient skin surface and the measurement point. Therefore, one set of TMR data can be used for all gantry angles because the dose characteristic is only dependent on depth of the isocentre inside the patient.

All modern radiotherapy is delivered isocentrically when more than a single field is used; this is especially important in rotational techniques where there is no possibility of moving the patient because the gantry is moved while the beam is on in one sweep. However, there remains one advantage of fixed SSD treatments that relate to the patient being further from the source of radiation, in order to use larger treatment fields. The primary example is the treatment of total body irradiation (TBI).

9.5 **Tissue inhomogeneity**

So far, consideration has only been given to the dose distribution within a homogeneous water phantom. However, in a patient, variations in tissues exist and these affect the dose distribution. For simple palliative treatments where machine parameters are calculated without a TPS one can ignore differences and assume water density throughout; but where greater accuracy is required, TPSs use tissue density to correct dose calculations.

For MV energy radiation it is *electron density* (number of electrons per unit volume) that dictates the attenuation of the primary photon beam and so dictates the kerma (section 5.1.3) at any point within the patient. A lower relative electron density, RED (to water) eg that in lung (0.15–0.3 typically) means that photons are less attenuated, i.e. a greater proportion of them travel through lung than they would through water of the same physical thickness. Bone RED on the other hand lies in the range 1.1–1.3 (depending on whether spongy or cortical) and is therefore more attenuating. In other words, for photon attenuation alone, 1cm of water is equivalent to approximately 4cm of lung or 0.8cm of bone.

These deviations from unity RED leads to the concept of equivalent path length. This is a simple method whereby one can multiply the physical distance traversed along the beam direction by the RED of the material in question. If this is repeated for all materials in the path and summed, then the total is termed the 'effective depth' or 'radiological path length' or 'radiological depth'.

There is a simple rule of thumb that says that (for far away from the inhomogeneity) for every 1cm of lung the downstream dose for a 6 MV beam is amplified by ~3% and for every 1cm of bone dose is diminished by ~2%. This effect of elongating or compressing isodoses can be seen distal (downstream) to the lung and bone inhomogeneities in Figure 9.11.

(a)   (b)   (c)

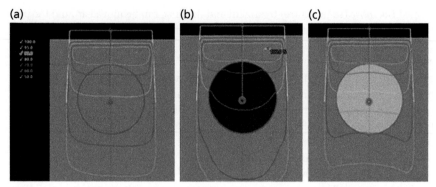

Figure 9.11 The effects on isodoses of tissues other than water. All fields 6MV and are set with identical field parameters. Dose at dmax is approximately 100% in all cases but the depth doses are heavily modified when the cylinder of water (a) is replaced by cylinder of lung equivalent (b) and a cylinder of cortical bone equivalent (c).

In reality, it is not only KERMA changes that determine absorbed dose because it is the electrons that give up their energy and then are absorbed by the medium, so the calculation of absorbed dose *inside* the heterogeneity and at *boundaries* of media with different densities is complex. Because of this complexity, how dose appears *in* or *very close to* inhomogeneities depends heavily on the sophistication of the calculation algorithm used for the calculation (see section 9.14).

Note in Figure 9.11 how the 95% isodose on the entrance lung surface is bowing around it back towards the surface whilst the lower isodoses are elongated.

9.6 **Bolus**

There are occasions when part of the target is close to the skin surface, such as in primary head and neck cancers or breast cancers with skin involvement. In these instances, the characteristic skin-sparing build-up effect of MV beam radiotherapy works against us and can lead to under-treatment of superficial disease.

To mitigate for this, some water-equivalent material (bolus) can be placed on the skin over the superficial target. This is usually between 5 mm and 10 mm thick and gives an additional layer in which build-up can occur, meaning that d_{max} occurs at or around the depth of the superficial target.

N.B. The presence of some essential pieces of equipment (e.g. the treatment couch and immobilization devices) are likely to provide a bolus effect when a radiation beam passes through them. This effect can be pronounced, potentially leading to high patient skin dose.

9.7 **Monitor unit calculations for simple plans**

9.7.1 **What is a monitor unit?**

Given the importance of accurate dose delivery to achieve the best tumour control with acceptable normal tissue complications, it might sound surprising to learn that the linac itself has no concept of absorbed dose nor its unit of Gray (Gy). Acknowledging this is the critical first step in understanding the importance of the 'monitor unit' (MU).

Monitor units are used by the linear accelerator as a 'count' of the number of radiation particles passing though the treatment head. The ionization chamber (also known as the monitor chamber) in the linac head (Figures 11.4 and 11.6) converts the free electrons created from ionization of air in the monitor chamber, as a result of radiation passing through it, to electrical charge which is recorded by the linac for each exposure.

The linac monitor chamber has no idea *where* the patient is in relation to the linac, nor does it know critical things like the depth of the target inside that patient. These parameters are for the radiotherapy team to decide, based on each individual case. Despite the linac not being able to determine dose directly, it is critical that members of the radiotherapy team *are* able to determine the dose inside the patient accurately for the bespoke set of parameters that we use for each individual patient (the treatment plan). There are a huge number of configurable parameters on linacs which affect the relationship between machine output *(monitor units)* and the patient *(absorbed dose)*.

The way we deal with this disconnect is to link MU and dose explicitly for a single set of linac parameters and at a specific point in the patient (or phantom). We call this set of rules and parameters the 'reference conditions' or 'calibration conditions'. This relationship is configurable by the physics team.

From this single reference condition we can use the relative correction factors (depth dose factor, output factor, wedge factor, etc.) to take us from that reference condition to patient plan condition. The reference condition is used in manual calculations of monitor units but is also required by the TPS in order to calculate dose correctly.

Being able to understand and use these correction factors in the appropriate way will both enable you to calculate MUs for simple beam arrangements and consolidate your knowledge of those linac parameters already discussed.

An example reference condition would be as follows:

- SSD = 100 cm
- Field size = 10 cm × 10 cm (at 100 cm SSD)
- Measurement point is at depth = d_{max} on the central axis

Under these specific conditions 1 MU will deliver 1 cGy to that point (Figure 9.13a)

The defined reference condition may be department specific.

9.7.2 The corrections

9.7.2.1 Correction for field size

Usually tumours are not square and nor do they demand a field size of 10 cm × 10 cm. Therefore, the first correction to make is for the field size in the patient condition. The field size changes two key beam factors for dose determination in the patient.

First, changes in field size affect the absolute dose per monitor unit delivered to d_{max}. This is called **output factor** (or field size factor or relative dose factor (section 6.6)). The larger the field size, the larger the scattered dose from the head of the machine (head or collimator scatter factor, Sc) and if the increase in field size translates to an increase in the volume of patient irradiated then this also increases the scattered dose to d_{max} from the patient themselves (phantom scatter factor, Sp).

Where the patient plan field is *larger* than the reference field we will be delivering a higher dose per MU at the reference point because of the increased scattered dose. Therefore, we will need *fewer* MUs than the reference condition to deliver the same dose. The converse is true of fields smaller than the reference field size.

Secondly, the change in field dimensions affect the relative depth dose curve (both PDD and TMR). The larger the field, the larger the relative amount of scattered radiation to the central axis inside the patient at depth beyond d_{max} compared with the dose at d_{max}.

At the time of machine commissioning (section 11.8.3), output factors and depth doses for a range of standard field shapes are typically measured. If we consider the number of potential field sizes with two independent collimators and all the potential shapes from multileaf collimators (MLCs), these are innumerable and not every possible combination can be measured directly. Therefore, we have a method to equate an 'equivalent' standard field size from all other potential field shapes in terms of the field's output factor and depth dose characteristics.

For simple rectangular fields we can use Day's Rule which says that a rectangular field of arbitrary side lengths a and b will be approximately equivalent to a square of side length a_{eq} where the area/perimeter ratio is maintained (Figure 9.12a).

$$Length\ of\ \text{side of equivalent square } a_{eq} = \frac{4(ab)}{2(a+b)} = \frac{2(ab)}{(a+b)}$$

For example, if a field size was 3 cm × 7 cm then the equivalent square side length would be:

$$a_{eq}\frac{2\times(7\times3)}{(7+3)} = \frac{42}{10} = 4.2\text{ cm}$$

This rule starts to break down where the aspect ratio of the rectangle, that is a:b, is more than 3:1, and so there are also tabulated data available to enable this correction. There are similar rules and tables for equivalent circles.

For more complex shapes than rectangles, for example where there is extensive shielding in the field, a more complex method is required to deduce the equivalent square. The most versatile is known as 'sector integration' or a Clarkson Integral whereby the open field aperture is split up into segments with the measuring point at the centre. If the field is divided up like a cake with each wedge having an equal angle of cut with its own radius to the aperture edge (Figure 9.12b), then each wedge can

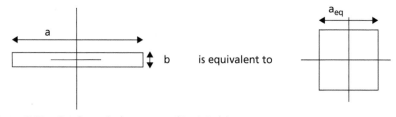

Figure 9.12a Simple equivalent square (Day's Rule).

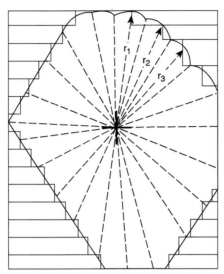

Figure 9.12b Complex Equivalent Square (Clarkson scatter integration calculation). The field is split into segments of equal angle. The radii of the first 3 segments (r1, r2 and r3) are shown.

be considered like a segment of a circular field of that radius. By knowing how much scatter would be received by that circular field component to its centre then adding this up for all segments and finally dividing through by the number of segments, you will come to an answer for the equivalent circle.

Hence, calculating the mean radius gives the radius of the equivalent circular field then the equivalent square can be calculated by multiplying the mean circular radius by 1.77.

9.7.2.2 Correction for depth

Tumours are not usually conveniently located at d_{max} and so a correction is required for depth inside the patient.

In the **fixed SSD patient plan**, if the calculation point is at depth d inside the patient, then we need to ensure that the inverse square law and the attenuation is taken into account in the correction from d_{max}, that is the source to reference point distance (SRPD) = 100 cm + d. This is exactly what PDD does.

In the **isocentric patient plan**, the source to axis is fixed (and the SSD varies instead). If the axis is used as the reference point, all fields have a SRPD = 100 cm. In this instance, to account for depth the only correction required between d_{max} and arbitrary depth d is for the attenuation for the material above the reference point. This is exactly what TMR does.

In both cases, we must ensure that we are using the correct depth dose curve for the correct equivalent size field, as determined above. In both cases we will always need to *increase* the number of MUs for any given dose at depth compared with delivering that dose to d_{max}. The amount we increase by is dictated by the relevant depth dose curve.

9.7.2.3 Correction for accessories

Anything else in the beam path between the source of radiation and the patient will have to be corrected for. The main one to consider is a wedge.

Wedges are very attenuating and can reduce radiation transmission by up to a factor of 4 compared with the equivalent open field. Treatment couches and patient immobilization accessories, which between them may require corrections of several percent also need to be accounted for.

9.7.3 'The' MU equation

To define one equation for the calculation of MUs is difficult. The reason it is difficult is that many of the factors can be defined and presented in different ways depending on the radiotherapy centre you áre working in.

For example, output factor could be defined as dose delivered (cGy) per MU, or indeed the number of MU to deliver 1 Gray. Wedge factors can be inverted depending on whether they are presented as transmission or attenuation factors. Sometimes depth dose factors are combined with output factors to give a combined factor.

And so, instead, it is vital to understand the effect of each of the differences between the reference condition and the patient plan condition so that you use the data you are presented with appropriately. This can be checked somewhat by ensuring that units on either side of the equation are balanced, however some quantities are unitless and so this method cannot be used on its own. The use of the equation also depends on whether the reference condition is fixed SSD or isocentric.

That said, here is a general equation for the calculation of MUs.

The definitions are:

♦ WF (wedge factor) as defined in section 6.5.2

♦ OF (output factor) is defined as dose per MU delivered (cGy/MU)

♦ TF (transmission factor) corrects for all other items in the beam path (e.g. treatment couch, immobilization equipment, etc.)

We assume here that the linac is calibrated in the 100 cm fixed SSD setting.

9.7.3.1 Fixed SSD treatment

$$MU = 100 \times Dose\ per\ fraction(Gy) \times \frac{100}{PDD} \times \frac{1}{OF(cGy/MU)} \times \frac{1}{TF} \times \frac{1}{WF}$$

9.7.3.2 Isocentric treatment

$$MU = 100 \times Dose\ per\ fraction(Gy) \times \frac{1}{TMR} \times \frac{1}{OF(cGy/MU)} \times \frac{1}{WF} \times \frac{1}{TF} \times \left(\frac{100}{100 + d_{max}}\right)^2$$

Points to note to explain these equations:

1) For both equations, we must convert dose in Gy (standard unit in the United Kingdom) to centigray (cGy) because we know that in the reference condition 1 MU will deliver 1 cGy to the reference point.

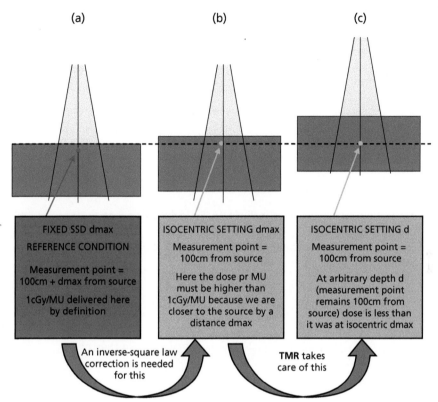

(a) (b) (c)

FIXED SSD dmax	ISOCENTRIC SETTING dmax	ISOCENTRIC SETTING d
REFERENCE CONDITION	Measurement point = 100cm from source	Measurement point = 100cm from source
Measurement point = 100cm + dmax from source	Here the dose pr MU must be higher than 1cGy/MU because we are closer to the source by a distance dmax	At arbitrary depth d (measurement point remains 100cm from source) dose is less than it was at isocentric dmax
1cGy/MU delivered here by definition		

An inverse-square law correction is needed for this

TMR takes care of this

Figure 9.13 An explanation for the inverse square law correction when calibrating at fixed SSD (a), calibrating isocentrically (b) and treating isocentrically (c). Dotted line indicates 100cm from the source of radiation.

2) PDD requires a further factor of 100 to convert the percentage to a ratio, whereas TMR is already a ratio and so does not require this.

3) Note that the units on each side of the equation balance.

4) Take a moment to check the equation works yourself by thinking about the reference condition and set the values in the fixed SSD equation yourself. You should see quite readily that if you wish to deliver 1 cGy, the number of MUs required is 1.

5) Note that an additional correction is required for the isocentric treatment scenario when the reference condition is fixed SSD. This is explained in Figure 9.13.

9.7.4 Worked examples

The following section contains some worked examples of MU calculations for simple arrangements. In each case we want to calculate the MU required per field per fraction. The data that you will require are tabulated below.

Worked example 1

Single field using 6 MV, 9 cm × 20 cm field size at 100 cm SSD. We want to deliver 8 Gy in 1 fraction to a point at 4 cm deep on the central axis

SSD = 100 cm, therefore we can use the fixed SSD equation.

$$MU = 100 \times Dose\ per\ fraction(Gy) \times \frac{100}{PDD} \times \frac{1}{OF(cGy/MU)} \times \frac{1}{TF} \times \frac{1}{WF}$$

Think about the differences to the reference condition:

1. Field size = 9 cm × 20 cm

We have output factor presented in Table 9.3. So looking up a 9 cm × 20 cm field dimension we can read off output factor of 1.009 cGy/MU

We must also calculate the equivalent square in order to use the correct depth dose data

$$a_{eq} = 2(ab)/(a + b) = 2 \times (9 \times 20)/(9 + 20) = 12.4\ cm$$

2. Depth, d = 4 cm

Now use the equivalent square to look up correct PDD (Table 9.1)

Table 9.1 6 MV PDD

Percentage Depth Dose, PDD 6 MV					
		Equivalent square field size (cm)			
		9	10	12	15
Depth (cm)	1	98.8	99.0	99.1	99.4
	1.5	100	100	100	100
	2	98.2	98.8	98.0	98.3
	3	93.9	94.6	94.1	94.5
	4	89.8	90.1	90.4	90.8
	5	85.3	85.8	86.3	86.8
	6	81.3	81.7	82.0	82.6
	7	77.2	77.7	78.1	78.7
	8	73.0	73.9	74.4	75.1
	9	69.3	70.0	70.6	71.5
	10	65.8	66.4	67.1	68.2

Looking along the horizontal row for depth of 4 cm and interpolate in the other direction between field sizes 12 cm and 15 cm for 12.4 cm equivalent square. This should bring you to a PDD value of 90.4% (1 dp).

3. Accessories

We aren't told of any and so we are in the same condition as the reference condition, therefore: TF = 1.00, WF = 1.00

Therefore the MUs required to deliver 8 Gy to 4 cm deep in this setting are:

$$MU = 100 \times 8Gy \times \frac{100}{90.4} \times \frac{1}{1.009\,cGy\,/\,MU} \times \frac{1}{1.00} \times \frac{1}{1.00} = 877\,MU$$

Note how the *larger* field size means that we needed *fewer MUs* because of the increased scatter compared with the reference condition and so we divide by a number greater than 1 for OF.

Note how the *increased depth* meant we needed *more MUs* compared with the reference condition

---

Worked example 2

95 cm SSD, 6 MV, 8 cm × 12 cm field size, to deliver 20 Gy in 5 fractions isocentrically to a point at 10 cm deep on the central axis.

SSD = 90 cm, depth = 10 cm, SSD + depth = 100 cm, therefore we must use isocentric equation:

$$MU = 100 \times Dose\ per\ fraction(Gy) \times \frac{1}{TMR} \times \frac{1}{OF(cGy\,/\,MU)} \times \frac{1}{WF} \times \frac{1}{TF} \times \left(\frac{100}{100 + d_{max}}\right)^2$$

Think about the differences to the reference condition:

1. Field size = 8 cm × 12 cm

We have output factor presented in Table 9.3. So looking up an 8 cm × 12 cm field dimension we can read off output factor of 0.992 cGy/MU

We must also calculate the equiv. square in order to use the correct depth dose data

$$a_{eq} = 2(ab)/(a + b) = 2 \times (8 \times 12)/(8 + 12) = 9.6\ cm$$

2. Depth, d = 10 cm

Use the equivalent square to look up correct TMR for this depth, energy, and field size (Table 9.2)

Table 9.2 6 MV TMR

Tissue Maximum Ratio, TMR 6 MV		Equivalent square field size (cm)				
		9	10	11	12	15
Depth (cm)	1.5	1.000	1.000	1.000	1.000	1.000
	2	0.997	0.997	0.997	0.997	0.997
	3	0.972	0.972	0.973	0.974	.977
	4	0.943	0.946	0.947	0.949	0.953
	5	0.916	0.917	0.918	0.921	0.930
	6	0.887	0.889	0.891	0.894	0.900
	7	0.857	0.861	0.864	0.868	0.874
	8	0.828	0.833	0.834	0.839	0.850
	9	0.798	0.803	0.805	0.809	0.821
	10	0.764	0.771	0.775	0.781	0.797

Looking along the horizontal row for depth of 10 cm and interpolate in the other direction between field sizes 9 cm and 10 cm for 9.6 cm equivalent square. This should bring you to a TMR value of 0.768 (3 dp).

3. Accessories

We aren't told of any wedge, therefore: TF = 1.00, WF = 1.00

Therefore the MUs required to deliver 4Gy per fraction (20 Gy in 5 f) to 10 cm deep in this setting are:

$$MU = 100 \times 4Gy \times \frac{1}{0.768} \times \frac{1}{0.992\,cGy\,/\,MU} \times \frac{1}{1.00} \times \frac{1}{1.00} \times \left(\frac{100}{100+1.5}\right)^2 = 502\,MU$$

Note how this time we needed the inverse square law correction to reduce the number of MUs because the calculation point is closer to the source than we would have been in the fixed SSD setting.

Also note how this time we had to increase the number of MUs by dividing by a number less than 1 for OF to account for the field size being smaller than the reference field size.

Where we are asked to calculate MUs for field arrangements with more than one field, we need to know the relative dose contribution expected from each field to the calculation point in order to do this. For equally weighted fields this is straightforward, we just divide the total dose required at the calculation point by the number of fields, for example. If we are delivering 8 Gy in a single fraction via two POP fields then we simply require 4 Gy from each field to the calculation point.

For unequally weighted fields, for example from a three-field plan where we wished to have a ratio of 40% from each lateral field with the remaining 20% from the posterior field, then we would have to calculate the field weighting in terms of dose first. So for an intended dose of 45 Gy in 25 fractions we would first calculate the total dose per fraction at 1.8 Gy then take the relative percentages of this to determine the intended dose per field, that is 40% × 1.8 Gy = 0.72 Gy from each lateral field and 0.36 Gy from the posterior field. The important thing to note is that all field weights must add up to 100%.

Worked example 3

Calculate the MUs required per field to deliver 30 Gy in 10 fractions to patient midplane via equally weighted, isocentric parallel-opposed fields. The patient separation is 20 cm with jaw settings of 15 cm × 15 cm; energy = 6 MV. Both fields have a 60-degree wedge applied.

Patient separation is 20 cm, therefore to set the isocentre in the middle of the patient, depth should be 10 cm (SSD = 100 − 10 cm) = 90 cm. We must use isocentric equation:

$$MU = 100 \times Dose\ per\ fraction(Gy) \times \frac{1}{TMR} \times \frac{1}{OF(cGy/MU)} \times \frac{1}{WF} \times \frac{1}{TF} \times \left(\frac{100}{100 + d_{max}}\right)^2$$

Think about the differences to the reference condition:

Table 9.3 6 MV Output Factors

Output factor (cGy/MU)					
	X(cm)				
		12	15	18	20
Y(cm)	8	0.992	0.997	1.000	1.001
	9	1.000	1.005	1.008	1.009
	10	1.010	1.012	1.013	1.015
	12	1.015	1.021	1.024	1.026
	15	1.021	1.032	1.042	1.045
	18	1.024	1.042	1.047	1.050
	20	1.026	1.045	1.050	1.054

Table 9.4 6 MV 60° Wedge Factors (EDW)

60 degree wedge factor (dynamic)				
	Square field dimension (cm)			
	5	10	15	20
Wedge factor	0.855	0.710	0.580	0.500

1. Field size = 15 cm × 15 cm

We have output factor presented in Table 9.3. So, looking up a 15 cm × 15 cm field dimension we can read off output factor of 1.032 cGy/MU

The field in this case is already square and so no equivalent square conversion needed.

2. Depth, d = 10 cm

Use the equivalent square to look up correct TMR for this depth, energy, and field size (Table 9.2)

Looking along the horizontal row for depth of 10 cm and 15 cm equivalent square field size. This should bring you to a TMR value of 0.797.

3. Accessories

There is a dynamic wedge in the field, this varies rapidly with field size, looking at Table 9.4, WF = 0.580; TF = 1.00

In this case the intended dose per field per fraction is 30 Gy/10 fractions × 50% = 1.5 Gy. Therefore the MUs required to deliver 1.5 Gy per field per fraction in this setting are:

$$MU = 100 \times 1.5\ Gy \times \frac{1}{0.797} \times \frac{1}{1.032\ cGy\,/\,MU} \times \frac{1}{0.580} \times \frac{1}{1.00} \times \left(\frac{100}{100+1.5}\right)^{2} = 305\,MU$$

Note this time the large change to the MU that the wedge brings about.

9.7.5 Top tips for MU calculations

Remember that you should always sense-check your answers because this equation presented here is *not universal* and will depend on the data that are given to you and how that data are presented.

It is very easy to insert the value on the top when it is meant to be underneath, etc. so you should think for each factor you are about to apply: 'Do I need more or fewer

MU than the reference condition?' and make sure the correction factor that you use is doing the right thing for you.

Also do a quick order of magnitude check. You know that at d_{max}, at around 100 cm SSD, 100 MU will give you about 1 Gy so to deliver 5 Gy you'll need about 500 MU at d_{max} and more at depth and more if you have a wedge.

9.8 Important definitions of volumes and dose

The International Commission on Radiation Units (ICRU) has produced several key reports which have steered the development of radiotherapy treatment planning since the early 1990s. These standardized the ways in which radiotherapy targets and organs at risk are defined and how radiation doses should be prescribed and reported. Their recommendations are not mandatory but are suggested for adoption to help useful comparison of clinical outcomes between different centres.

9.8.1 What is the ICRU?

The ICRU was formed in 1925. This group of volunteers' primary objective was to propose an internationally agreed upon unit for the measurement of radiation as applied to medicine. The group now publishes guidance on a wide range of radiation issues including volume and dose definition.

They have produced a series of reports to describe 'clear, well- defined, unambiguous, and universally accepted concepts and terminology ... to ensure a common understanding' and therefore ensure 'a useful exchange of information between different centres'.

In 1978 they produced a report ICRU 29 'Dose Specification for Reporting External Beam Therapy with Photons and Electrons'. As technology advanced, they subsequently published ICRU 50 in 1993 and then ICRU 62 in 1999 to keep up with developing techniques. There were additional reports recommending dose prescribing and reporting for intensity modulated radiotherapy (IMRT) (ICRU 83) in 2010 and similarly for stereotactic radiotherapy (ICRU 91) in 2019.

Although the ICRU reports are guidance and not statutory documents, they are avidly followed worldwide.

9.8.2 Volume definition

To treat a patient with cancer with radiotherapy, at a minimum we need to be able to identify which regions of the body we want to direct the radiation at (the targets) and which parts to avoid. There are many ways this can be done, however it makes sense if there is an international consensus on naming and volume definitions. This has many advantages, allowing comparison of treatments between different departments and countries.

The volumes defined can be split into the following categories:

- Malignant disease
  - Gross Tumour Volume (GTV)
  - Clinical Target Volume (CTV)
  - Planning Target Volume (PTV)

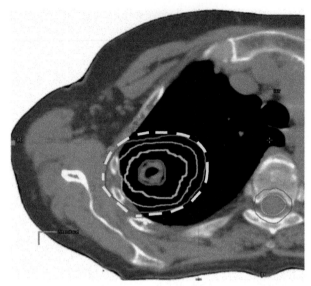

Figure 9.14 Lung tumour showing GTV (blue), CTV (cyan), ITV (green), PTV (red), treated volume (yellow dotted line), OAR (spinal cord, yellow line), PRV (magenta).

- Treated Volume
- Organs at Risk
- Irradiated Volume

First let's consider the malignant disease definitions; these can be thought of as concentric circles in 2D or spheres in reality, increasing in volume (Figure 9.14).

9.8.2.1 GTV

The GTV is the 'gross demonstrable extent and location of the malignant growth' that is the tumour. The GTV may also be extended to encompass metastatic lymph spread. So, we need to make sure that the GTV is always in the treatment beam!

However, there may in some cases be no GTV; for example if it has been removed by surgery.

9.8.2.2 CTV

The CTV includes all of the GTV (if present) and any subclinical malignant spread, that is all of the cancer. This is the volume that must be fully treated, that is it should always be in the treated dose region if one is to achieve the aim of radical radiotherapy.

Both the GTV and CTV are volumes that one could mark on the patient if the disease was only skin deep. As the patient moves, the CTV moves because it is all part of the patient. This is an important point, because as the CTV moves with the patient, we consider it from the patient's point of view. It is called being in the patient's 'frame of reference'. However, the CTV can also move with the organ it is in, for example lung cancer. Hold on to this thought, we'll come on to moving CTVs soon!

9.8.2.3 PTV

Now, the GTV and CTV are patient volumes, but we are aiming to treat them with an external beam treatment unit. For this example, we'll use a linac. Unfortunately, linacs are not perfect machines. From day to day there will be small differences in how they operate due to mechanical imperfections. Additionally, as the patient lies on the couch each day, even with very good immobilization, there will be small differences in their position (we are looking for millimetre accuracy).

The patient will be treated on many days and we want to make sure that the CTV is in the high dose region, each time the patient is treated. As such, we need to take account of all the variables that can affect the accuracy of the treatment delivery. Put simply, we combine all these together: patient setup variation, likely CTV movement, linac mechanical variations, etc., and deduce a safety margin to increase the CTV by. By increasing the CTV by this amount we create the PTV. The aim is that by irradiating the PTV we will always be irradiating the CTV. It is worth noting that if the CTV is close to the skin surface the PTV may actually extend outside of the patient.

The size and shape of the PTV dictate how the linac will be set to treat the CTV. As such, it is linked to the linac, not to the patient. The PTV is a region in space around the linac isocentre. The technical (ICRU) speak for this is that the CTV and GTV are in the 'patient frame of reference' and the PTV is in the 'linac frame of reference'.

The PTV is an often-misunderstood volume, it is not linked to the patient as such. If you consider the CTV (for a moment) as a basketball, then the PTV is analogous to the hoop!

As we mentioned, we need to irradiate a larger volume than the CTV (the PTV) to be sure of always treating the CTV. As you may have noticed, the day-to-day variations that affect the CTV could be split into two main groups: those that are due to the patient's internal anatomy and those external to the patient. This subtlety is addressed in ICRU 62, with two additional margins defined to help classify the contributions to the total margin added to the CTV to create the PTV. These are the internal margin and the setup margin.

9.8.2.4 ITV

The CTV shape can be influenced by adjacent organs, for example bladder and rectum filling both impact on prostate location and shape. This change in CTV size/shape is assigned a label in ICRU language as the internal margin (IM). If we add the IM to the CTV we get the internal target volume (ITV). The ITV is meant to encompass the CTV as it varies with the patient's internal anatomy.

9.8.2.5 SM

The setup margin (SM) encompasses all the other factors that could lead to the CTV being missed by the treatment field. These are factors that are external to the patient. As such, they are considered relative to the linac. This can be reduced by good patient immobilization and/or use of online correction.

These two additional volumes give us the following sequence:

Patient-centred volumes: GTV → CTV + IM → ITV
Treatment-centred volumes: ITV + SM → PTV

There is nothing complex about these two extra margins, they are merely added to help clarify where the data come from to justify the growth of CTV to PTV.

9.8.2.6 Treated volume (TV)

In most cases this is the volume of the 95% isodose. Using modern treatment techniques like VMAT, the TV is generally approximately the same size as the PTV. Using simpler techniques, it is usually larger.

9.8.2.7 Organs at risk (OAR)

All tissue outside in the CTV is 'normal tissue' and the dose to this should be kept as low as possible. However, not all normal tissue is equally sensitive. Organs that are known to be especially radiation sensitive are usually outlined in the TPS as OAR. Normal tissue tolerance levels need to be considered when prescribing radiotherapy, based on normal tissue complication probabilities (NTCPs, see section 15.3.1) and clinical evidence.

9.8.2.8 PRV

The OAR move with the patient and are susceptible to the same random and systematic errors as the CTV. As such, we grow the OAR volume by a set amount to create the planning organ at risk volume (PRV). Consider this a safety margin around the sensitive structure.

9.8.2.9 PTV meets PRV

There may be times where the PTV and PRV(s) overlap. At this point it is up to the clinician to decide which volume takes priority if there is a conflict between the intended prescription dose for the PTV and dose tolerance for the PRV.

9.8.2.10 Irradiated volume

This is simply quoted as the volume of tissue that receives a dose that is considered significant in relation to normal tissue tolerance.

9.8.3 Dose reporting (and where do we prescribe to?)

A radiotherapy treatment plan generates a *lot* of dose data and the question arises as to how to characterize or define the dose to the volume of interest, the PTV.

ICRU Report 50 introduced the concept of the ICRU Reference Point.

The ICRU defines this point as:

1) The dose at the point should be clinically relevant;
2) The point should be easy to define in a clear and unambiguous way;
3) The point should be selected so that the dose can be accurately determined;
4) The point should be in a region where there is no steep dose gradient.

Ideally, the ICRU reference point should be on the isocentre which should be in the centre of the PTV. However, this is not always possible. As a minimum, the reference point should be in the PTV and conform to the four criteria above.

The dose at the ICRU Reference Point is, with some degree of inevitability, defined as the ICRU Reference Dose.

As a minimum, according to ICRU50/62, one should report the:

♦ Dose to the ICRU reference point;

♦ Maximum dose to the PTV (ideally this should also be the maximum patient dose);

♦ Minimum dose to the PTV.

It is possible to produce a lot more information than this about a treatment plan. Indeed, for advanced treatments, such as IMRT or VMAT, one would need more information to judge if a plan was suitable for patient treatment! As such, dose volume histograms (DVHs) are produced (section 9.12.2). These, in conjunction with the 3D dose distribution, help to decided what is an acceptable plan, and form the record of the patient's treatment.

ICRU Reports 50 and 62 recommend that, in general, the PTV be covered by the 95% isodose, with the maximum less than 107%. This is commonly interpreted as 95 to 105% covering the PTV for conventional radiotherapy. Note that for stereotactic radiotherapy where dose heterogeneity is not seen as a detrimental effect, and is sometimes actually welcomed, there are different recommendations; these are discussed later.

ICRU Report 83 suggested that for highly conformal treatment delivery, the dose should be reported to a volume rather than a point. The report suggested that the median dose be used—the dose covering 50% of the PTV, also called the D50%—though in practice the mean dose to the PTV may also be used. This report also introduced the PTV 'near dose minimum' and 'near dose maximum'. Rather than being points, it was suggested that these should be volumes. The dose minimum is the dose covering 98% of the PTV, D98%, and the dose maximum is the dose covering 2% of the PTV, D2%. The near dose maximum concept is also use for OARs.

The purpose of a dose prescription is to turn relative dose (in percentages) shown on the treatment plan into absolute dose in Gray (Gy). It also enables calculation of treatment monitor units. (Note that in some centres, TPS calculations can be done in absolute dose rather than relative dose.)

For simple planning, a single point in the relative (percentage) distribution is chosen (usually on the 100% isodose) and this is assigned to the prescribed dose. Now all the percentage isodoses can be expressed in Gy. This point is called the ICRU reference point, and is reported along with dose volume data, and the median dose to the PTV.

For more complex, IMRT/VMAT plans, the prescription is to a volume—usually the mean or median PTV dose.

9.9 Treatment planning systems

A TPS is a complex set of software and hardware used to generate radiotherapy treatment plans and associated data for transfer to a linac (see Chapter 4). A TPS is needed for anything more complex than those described in section 9.3. CT has long been the patient imaging modality of choice for modelling the patient because it has very accurate spatial information and robust conversion of Hounsfield units to electron (or mass) density for calculating dose in heterogeneous media. However, CT has its drawbacks in terms of soft-tissue contrast and so more recently MRI-only planning has become possible with the use of appropriate conversions to electron density and MRI sequences that allow for full acquisition of the patient whilst minimizing inherent geometric distortions present in MRI (see Chapter 8).

9.9.1 Defining volumes

The imaging modality chosen is used to define GTV and CTV and OARs. TPSs have various drawing tools available to allow you to indicate these volumes in 3D on the virtual patient anatomy. Generation of PTVs from expansion of CTV is possible automatically either uniformly or not. Care must be taken at this stage as any errors may impact on the clinical outcome. A similar volume growing process is carried out with the OAR, some of which are grown to make PRVs.

9.9.2 The beam's eye view (BEV) and digitally reconstructed radiograph (DRR)

Planning systems offer a feature called a beam's eye view (BEV) which allows visualization of the patient as if you were looking from the X-ray source in the treatment head. In this BEV one can switch patient structures on or off (e.g. body contour, PTV, OAR) and collimator and MLC positions can be visualized directly. This can be useful for field shaping in conformal radiotherapy and to ensure optimal selection of gantry, collimator, and floor angles with respect to PTV and PRV(s). In Figure 9.15 note how

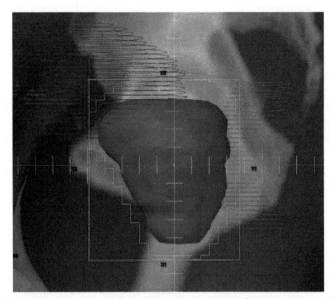

Figure 9.15 BEV showing PTV (red), bladder (blue) and MLC field edges (yellow), overlayed on a DRR.

the MLC is not fitted exactly to the PTV. This in intentional, as remember that the beam edge is defined by the 50% isodose and so to achieve coverage of dose with the 95% isodose, the field border has to be a number of millimetres beyond the PTV edge in the BEV.

BEVs almost always incorporate a digitally reconstructed radiograph (DRR). This is where the 3D data from the primary imaging modality are re-projected from the point of the observer using divergent ray-lines through the CT set such that it emulates a classic plain X-ray. Information is superimposed in 2D but this can be used to verify patient position on treatment by comparing with a kV or MV image (section 10.2.1).

9.9.3 The difference between forward and inverse planning

3D conformal treatments are usually forward planned, that is the planner decides on all the treatment parameters (field size, beam weight, gantry angle, etc.) then calculates the plan to see what the dose distribution looks like. If this is not optimal then they change one (or many) parameters and recalculate based on that input change. This is an iterative process by the planner and is adequate for simple beam modulation options: field size, field weight, and wedging.

Inverse planning is the opposite of this iterative process, in this case the planner sets requirements or criteria for the required plan. For example, the planner might require that at least 98% of the PTV is covered by 95% of the prescription dose. An optimization algorithm will then attempt to find a solution using a large range of options. When an acceptable solution is found by the algorithm, the computer then generates maps of photon fluence for the linac to deliver and computes the linac parameters required to generate that fluence.

Note: 'inverse planning' should not be confused with 'reverse planning'. Reverse planning means that where there is a conflict between PTV and PRV doses, the PTV dose is compromised by just enough to the balance point such that the PRV dose tolerance is upheld, for example setting an absolute maximum dose to spinal cord in a head and neck treatment, then compromising PTV coverage to attain this.

9.10 Intensity modulated radiotherapy (IMRT)

An open radiation field can be said to be of (almost) uniform intensity. If we want to create more complex distributions we need to modify the radiation dose coming through different parts of the field. The simplest type of intensity modulation is by the use of a wedge. This can be thought of as 1D modulation. However, to create curved isodose distributions (to bend round spinal cord, for example) we need to be able to modulate the radiation field in 2D. This is achieved by creating sub-field shapes using the MLC to effectively create lots of 2D modulations. Each opposing pair of MLC leaves work together to create a strip of modulated dose. If the leaves are closed, then nearly no dose gets through (so we can create an area of very low dose), as the leaves are opened more radiation gets through. So the size of the gap between the leaves dictates how much radiation gets to each part of the treatment field (Figure 9.16). If

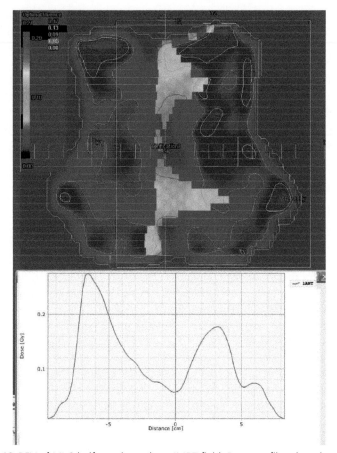

Figure 9.16 BEV of MLC halfway through an IMRT field. Dose profile taken through vertical axis.

we have 80 or more pairs of leaves moving across the radiation field together, we can create very complex radiation dose distributions.

- IMRT can be delivered through a series of sub-fields with the gantry in the same position before changing gantry angle and repeating. This is known as step-and-shoot IMRT.
- It can also be delivered by moving the MLC whilst the beam is on at each fixed gantry angle, this is known as dynamic IMRT (Figure 9.16).
- To increase the degree of modulation available further we can also move the MLCs and gantry whilst the beam is on whilst also varying gantry rotation speed and dose rate. This is known as volumetric modulated arc therapy (VMAT). This method, with its extra degree of potential parameters to change, can offer equally complex dose distributions compared with IMRT in a significantly shorter delivery time.

9.11 **Stereotactic radiotherapy**

Stereotactic means 'defining precise positioning in space' and grew out of neurosurgical techniques developed by a neurophysiologist Victor Horsley and mathematician Robert Clarke in the early twentieth century. Using cranial topographic knowledge along with an external frame of reference that was rigidly connected to the skull, an internal target could be navigated to precisely by surgical tools in a relatively non-invasive way compared with open neurosurgery.

Those early surgical tools were eventually replaced with a kV X-ray source in the mid-twentieth century (coining the term 'radiosurgery') and then the kV source was replaced with a series of cobalt-60 sources which had the benefit of using megavoltage energy gamma rays for deep-seated targets. This device became known as the GammaKnife and used frame-based technology alongside pre-treatment MRI to define the frame of reference position with respect to the target. This technology is still used today but is limited to intracranial indications.

Stereotactic radiosurgery (SRS) is generally characterized by the following:

◆ Sub-millimetre geometric targeting accuracy

◆ Very sharp and well-defined dose gradients beyond the PTV periphery

◆ Extremely high fractional doses, which are ablative in nature (hence sometimes being thought of as a surgical tool)

◆ High degrees of dose heterogeneity within the target (the dose in the centre of the tumour can be up to double that at the edge of the PTV). Dose prescription is at the edge rather than near the centre of the PTV

Linac manufacturers have achieved these benefits using a 'conventional' accelerator. This has extended the application of SRS beyond dedicated devices and to treatment sites outside the skull. High-quality imaging has replaced the invasive rigid fixation devices; similarly high levels of coincidence with the treatment system are maintained.

It is worth spending a moment on the naming system used here to clarify similar (and sometimes overlapping) terms. All four terms below can be easily interchanged with the more generic term **extremely hypofractionated radiotherapy.**

Stereotactic radiosurgery (SRS): the largest dose single fraction intracranial treatments that are likely to be ablative in nature.

Stereotactic radiotherapy (SRT): multi-fraction intracranial treatment that may or may not be ablative in nature.

Stereotactic ablative body radiotherapy (SABR) is a term that originated in the United States, originally used to describe treating primary lung cancer ablatively but now used for many extracranial indications.

Stereotactic body radiotherapy (SBRT) is the term that originated in the United Kingdom that is used interchangeably with 'SABR' but removes the term 'ablative' and so explicitly allows for a downwards extension of the dose per fraction range.

Conventionally fractionated radiotherapy delivers doses of around 2 Gy per fraction over a protracted period, which exploits the inherent radiobiological differences

(a)

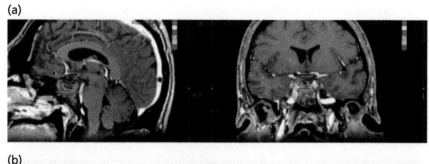

(b)

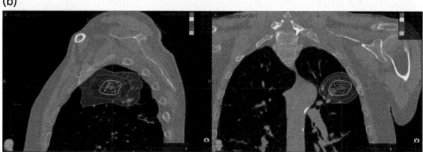

Figure 9.17 (a) Stereotactic treatment of a residual pituitary adenoma, prescription 25 Gy in a single fraction. Note the peripheral prescription dose (yellow) and its conformity to the PTV (red contour) with the substantially higher doses inside the PTV. Note also the very steep dose gradient to the optic pathway PRV (green contour) a little over 2 mm from the PTV edge at closest point. To maintain the optic pathway tolerance of 10 Gy with almost full target coverage, the dose gradient required here is ~6 Gy per mm (25% / mm). (b) Stereotactic treatment of a primary lung cancer, prescription dose 54 Gy in 3 fractions. Note the 54 Gy peripheral dose (yellow) and its conformity to the PTV (red contour) with the majority of the ITV (green contour) receiving more than 68 Gy. Note how the steep dose gradients mean that the volume of lung that receives more than 12.5 Gy is minimized.

between the tumour and the surrounding OAR(s). However, the lower end of the extreme hypofractionation spectrum used in stereotactic radiotherapy starts at 5–6 Gy per fraction (delivered over 3–8 fractions). This dose per fraction could be used, for example, in the pelvic re-irradiation setting or in the more centrally positioned primary lung cancer setting.

At the other end of the dose-per-fraction spectrum however, doses up to 25 Gy in a single fraction are used for small intracranial metastatic disease or pituitary adenoma (Figure 9.17), escalating further up to 60–90 Gy in a single fraction for the treatment of trigeminal neuralgia. Extracranially, 54 Gy in three fractions in used the treatment of small early-stage peripheral primary lung cancers, with some institutions more recently routinely using single fraction doses of 30–34 Gy in this setting.

These much higher fractional doses can be delivered without the risk of intolerable sequalae due to the following characteristics of stereotactic radiotherapy.

- **Treating only patients with a relatively small volume of disease burden.** Smaller gross tumour volume (GTV) means that treatment volumes are minimized which minimizes dose to the surrounding normal tissue.

- **Using precise tumour localization methods.** Using sophisticated methods of patient immobilization, motion-management, and imaging & correction strategies mean that internal margins (IM) and setup margins (SM) can be minimized. These strategies in turn minimize PTV which minimize dose to surrounding normal tissue. Motion management techniques are discussed further below.

- **Delivering dose distributions with very steep dose gradients** beyond the PTV edge (typically 10–25% of prescription dose per mm). This is typically done by increasing the number of beams and increasing the solid angle over which beams are delivered. When the beam central axis does not remain in the same axial plane throughout its delivery, this is termed a non-coplanar approach and can improve dose gradients markedly in the axial plane, making dose distributions more isotropic in three dimensions.

9.11.1 Motion management techniques

The aim of motion management is to reduce the internal margin (IM) and fall into these broad categories:

- **tumour tracking** where the tumour or its surrogate (e.g. implanted fiducial markers) and its motion are visualized or modelled in near real-time such that the beam aperture 'follows' the tumour motion whilst the beam is on.

- **abdominal compression** uses external physical compression of the diaphragm/abdomen to restrict breathing motion to a tolerable level. This can be used alongside gating or standalone.

- **active breathing control** is akin to abdominal compression but restricts the respiratory motion by limiting the patient's air intake using a controlled respirator. This can be used alongside gating or standalone.

- **gating** where the target motion is assessed on the treatment unit using the tumour itself or an on-treatment surrogate alongside knowledge of the respiratory pattern from pre-treatment imaging. The treatment beam is on for only a sub-part of the respiratory cycle chosen by the treatment planning team usually where the target least mobile.

9.11.2 Stereotactic technology

In addition to the extra care taken to minimize SM and IM and improve dose gradients, the other main differences between conventionally fractionated radiotherapy and stereotactic radiotherapy are that flattening filter-free (FFF, section 11.3.2.3) beams tend to be used. There are two reasons for this, first the dose rate can be increased significantly because the physical filter is removed from the primary photon path. Increased dose rates minimize treatment times and are particularly useful when treating mobile tumours using motion-management techniques. Secondly, FFF beams are heavily peaked in intensity towards the central axis and allow for increased internal dose compared with the edge of the field. This is usually seen as an advantage in stereo-tactic radiotherapy (or at least, not a detriment).

Linear accelerator technologies that can now facilitate stereotactic radiotherapy delivery include:

Accuray CyberKnife® uses planar kV stereoscopic imaging coupled with non-isocentric, multiple small fixed-collimation or IMRT fields from a single energy accelerator mounted on a robotic arm. Specializes in dose conformity for the smallest intracranial lesions and real-time tracking for mobile extracranial lesions using semi-predictive modelling but does not yet have CT imaging.

Varian and **Elekta** linacs typically use cone beam computed tomography (CBCT) coupled with non-coplanar arcs or non-coplanar VMAT to exploit beam delivery angles. The benefits being that the linacs are widely available and versatile. **Viewray MRIdian®** and **Elekta Unity** use 3D and 4D magnetic resonance (MR) imaging and so specialize in soft tissue target localization, motion tracking, and plan adaptation. However, delivery is not currently available with volumetric arcs and is restricted to a co-planar approach due to the design of the MR unit.

Additional ancillary technologies can further improve intra-fractional target localization assurance whilst delivering the larger doses per fraction. The main examples of these technologies are surface-guided radiotherapy using the external patient anatomy as a surrogate of target position and external stereoscopic kV imaging systems that can be used to define internal bony anatomy or fiducial marker position.

9.12 Plan verification and evaluation

9.12.1 Isodose display

When the calculation is complete, the TPS computer will link together regions of equal dose, called isodoses. These are analogous to contour lines of equal height on a map. When a TPS performs a calculation, it is actually calculating dose to a 3D series of points called a dose grid which covers the patient anatomy treated. Isodoses are interpolated from dose grid points but the doses to individual grid points can be used to generate dose volume histograms (DVHs), a valuable plan assessment and comparison tool.

9.12.2 Dose volume histograms

A DVH is a 2D graphical representation of the 3D dose distribution for individual organs. It is useful for evaluating and comparing treatment plans. However, DVHs do not replace the full isodose distribution as they do not contain geometric information: they can tell you the volume of tissue receiving a certain dose but not tell you where in the OAR or PTV the dose is.

There are two types of DVH in use in radiotherapy.

- Differential (frequency) DVH

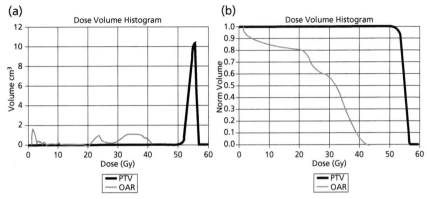

Figure 9.18 DVHs showing PTV and OAR data. (a) is a differential DVH, (b) is an integral DVH.

- volume (v_i) of organ receiving a dose (D_i)
- Integral (cumulative) DHV
- volume (v_i) of organ receiving a dose (D_i) *or greater*

The differential DVH shows the homogeneity of dose to a structure (Figure 9.18a). In the case of a PTV one could look at the width of the peak (narrow is good) and the maximum and minimum doses are easy to see. However, this DVH is not so useful for OAR.

The integral DVH is the one most used to give PTV and OAR data (Figure 9.18b). The two most common uses of this DVH are to see the:

1) global maximum received by an organ (serial organs), such as spinal cord maximum.

2) dose received by a certain volume of an organ (parallel organs), such as V20 of lung.

Data can be displayed in a DVH in absolute or relative form. In both examples above, the dose is shown as absolute in Gy. In the differential DVH, the volume is absolute in cm³. In the integral case, it is in relative or fractional format.

9.12.3 Stereotactic radiotherapy plan assessment

There are some specific metrics that are used to evaluate stereotactic radiotherapy plans.

9.12.3.1 Conformity Index

This is the metric that numerically describes how well the prescription dose conforms to the PTV shape or, conversely, how much 'spillage' of prescription dose there is beyond the PTV. There are a number of similar metrics used but perhaps the best known two are the Radiation Therapy Oncology Group (RTOG) conformity index and Paddick Conformity Index.

$$CI_{RTOG} = \frac{PIV}{PTV} \qquad CI_{Paddick} = \left(\frac{PTV_{PIV}}{PIV}\right)\left(\frac{PTV_{PIV}}{PTV}\right) = \left(\frac{PTV_{PIV}}{PIV}\right) \times coverage$$

PIV = prescription isodose volume, that is the volume of the patient that contains the prescription isodose

PTV = planning target volume, that is the volume to which one is trying to conform the prescription isodose to

PTV_{PIV} = the volume of PTV that receives the prescription isodose

Coverage = the proportion of the PTV that contains the prescription isodose, expressed as a ratio

CI_{RTOG} is the simplest index and measures the similarity of the PIV and the PTV physical volumes. The ideal ratio would be unity with decreasing plan quality in terms of prescription dose over spillage as the index rises above 1 and decreasing plan quality indicating target under-coverage as the index deviates significantly below 1. However, because this metric simply uses PIV and PTV in the equation it is not sophisticated enough to detect if the PIV and PTV were in different locations or completely different shapes that happened to have the same physical volume. The values of this metric clearly depend on technology employed and the complexity of the PTV shape, but broadly speaking, plan values might lie in the range 0.95–1.30.

$CI_{Paddick}$ rectifies these flaws by instead computing the (inverse) ratio of the PIV to the amount of PTV that is receiving that prescription isodose (hence being able to detect when the target and the isodose are in different locations), then multiplies this quantity by the coverage. $CI_{Paddick}$ has a maximal (and ideal) value of unity with decreasing plan quality shown by decreasing value towards zero. By using coverage in the index, this allows for fairer comparison of plans where coverage values vary between them. This metric obviously depends on technology employed and the complexity of the PTV shape but broadly plan values might lie in the range 0.70–0.98.

Some systems use an inverse $CI_{Paddick}$ as this seems more intuitive because it is more akin to the pre-existing CI_{RTOG} whilst maintaining the added sophistication of the Paddick terms.

9.12.3.2 Gradient index (GI)

This is akin to conformity index but is addressing the intermediate dose spillage. There are fewer metrics of this type and the most used is the simplest:

$$GI = \frac{Volume\ of\ patient\ receiving\ 50\%\ of\ prescription\ dose}{Volume\ of\ patient\ receiving\ prescription\ dose}$$

The smaller this ratio is, the more tightly packed are the isodoses between prescription dose and half of prescription dose meaning a faster falling dose gradient between those two levels. This metric obviously depends on technology employed and the complexity of the plan (including surrounding organs at risk), the tissue type in which the target resides and the size of the PTV but broadly planned values might lie in the range 3.0–7.0.

9.13 **Checking of individual patient plans**

9.13.1 Conformal

A physics check of a conformal plan should at a minimum confirm that the patient details are all correct; the moves from tattoos to treatment centre are correct; the plan is a 'good plan' (i.e. dose distribution covers PTV and avoids PRV); plan is for the correct dose and fractionation, all local processes have been followed, and (finally) that the MUs are correct. The MU check should be a fully independent calculation of the MU required to deliver the prescribed dose to the prescription point in the patient.

9.13.2 **IMRT/VMAT**

The checks above are all necessary for these more complex plans, however there is an additional test done due to an extra risk factor that these treatments have. IMRT plans require the MLC to move during treatment and what the TPS shows is an interpretation of how the TPS thinks the MLC will work. The resultant dose distribution in the patient is totally dependent not only on the MLC working correctly, but also on the TPS algorithm modelling the unique leaf motion for this patient correctly. As such, all patient IMRT/VMAT plans are verified in a specialist software system, or measured on a linac. This is discussed further in section 15.4.3.

9.14 **Dose calculation models**

9.14.1 **What exactly are we trying to model?**

Scientists have worked for over 50 years to develop dose calculation methods that more closely represented the true nature of dose deposition in patients. Remember, photons interact with electrons and electrons deposit energy, which is dose. The goal is to model dose deposition accurately, taking into account patient shape and different tissue types. All algorithm developments are further attempts to calculate the electronic equilibrium problem described in section 5.2.3.

All treatment planning dose models (algorithms) are an approximation of what is actually going on in the patient. From what you learned about photon and electron interactions, you already know more than you think about how the entire process takes place.

Essentially, high energy photons (primary radiation beam) interact with matter creating a slightly lower energy photon and a moving electron broken free from its atom (both are 'scatter') with the photon going on to liberate more electrons, etc. All these electrons move through the material/tissue losing energy to other electrons (scatter) causing 'dose' to be deposited. Everything we are discussing here is trying to model this process. It is the electrons we are most interested in because they deposit dose. So, how do we model photon interactions with electrons—and what happens to them after the interaction? The closest to reality is a technique called 'Monte Carlo' modelling, discussed later. However, simpler and quicker calculation methods are available, which we will discuss first.

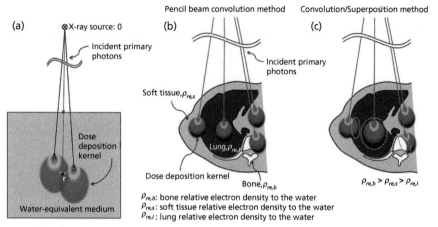

Figure 9.19 (a) Photons hitting small volume of water give resultant dose shown as ellipses. Dose intensity decreases with distance. (b) Dose deposition kernels applied to a CT scan. (c) Shows the scaling of the kernels due to different tissue densities. The dotted regions indicate where scaling will take place.

Adapted with permission from Radiology Key, 'Visualization of Dose Distributions for Photon Beam Radiation Therapy During Treatment Delivery'. Available at https://radiologykey.com/visualization-of-dose-distributions-for-photon-beam-radiation-therapy-during-treatment-delivery/

9.14.2 Dose kernels

Before we go further, we need to discuss dose kernels. A kernel is simply a computer-generated map of the dose that will arise in surrounding tissue for a tiny radiation beam (e.g. 6 MV) hitting a small volume of water, the interaction point. This is a map of the energy deposited by electrons generated after photon interactions in the small volume of water. The dose falls off the further you get from the interaction point. A kernel looks bit like an asymmetric ellipse, elongated in the direction of travel of the radiation beam (Figure 9.19).

These are created in advance, usually during the commissioning of a planning system. They are calculated once (using Monte Carlo modelling, section 9.14.4) and then used for each patient calculation. Therefore, potentially time-consuming calculations can be taken out of the planning path.

One dose kernel by itself is not much use and we need to add many of them together to produce a dose distribution for a single beam—a bit like using Lego. A typical radiotherapy plan will consist of many small volumes of tissue, each of which will release energy and deposit dose in surrounding small volumes of tissue. Obviously, the energy released in each volume needs to be modified according to the intensity of the beam at that point in the patient (i.e. accounting for depth and lateral profile shape). The processes of adding all the kernels together are known mathematically as either convolution or superposition, hence the names convolution or superposition dose models.

9.14.3 Convolution vs superposition?

In a completely homogenous medium, like water, convolution and superposition dose models behave pretty much the same. Unfortunately, patients are not completely homogenous.

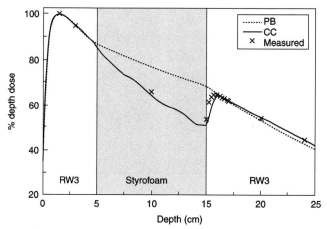

Figure 9.20 Graph showing how %DD through lung (styrofoam) and plastic water (RW3) are calculated by convolution pencil beam (PB) algorithm and superposition algorithm (CC) versus measurement.

Reproduced with permission from A. Nisbet, I. Beange, H. Vollmar, C. Irvine, A. Morgan & D. Thwaites (2004). Dosimetric verification of a commercial collapsed cone algorithm in simulated clinical situations. *Radiotherapy & Oncology*, **73**, 1: 79–88, with permission of British Institute of Radiology.

Historically, convolution dose models were available first. They appeared in the 1990s and represented a significant development at the time. They were, though, limited by the way they dealt with tissue heterogeneity.

The classic example is radiation passing through lung (Figure 9.20). The convolution model scales the kernels along the path of the beam, but not laterally. In this sense, they only model the heterogeneity along a line and are known as 1D models.

Variations of the superposition algorithm go by such names as 'collapsed cone' or 'AAA' depending on the manufacturer. The main difference is that these algorithms can correct for tissue inhomogeneity in all directions. They are truly 3D. They model the loss of scattered radiation in lung, the build-up of scatter (and dose) upon re-entering tissue after lung and the broadening of the beam penumbra in lung (Figures 9.20 and 9.21). This is done by scaling the dose kernels, roughly in proportion to the densities of the materials they are passing through. The superposition type models are generally accepted to be an accurate type of dose calculation model currently and can model missing tissue and the effects of differing tissue density on radiation beams. Figures 9.19b and 9.19c show the very basic principles of superposition and how dose scaling can be applied according to tissue density. There will be many more kernels than those shown here!

9.14.4 Monte Carlo

Monte Carlo calculations are considered the 'gold standard' in terms of dose calculation and have been used as a benchmark for new dose models that appear. Due to advances in computer processor power, Monte Carlo calculations are now starting to become available in the clinic for both photon and electron beams.

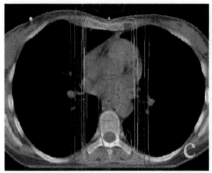
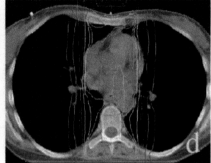

Figure 9.21 The same patient treatment calculated with pencil beam, c, and superposition, d. The more accurate modelling of scatter in d can be seen by the low dose levels (blue lines) spreading laterally, but the high dose lines (green and orange) being drawn in medially.

Reproduced with permission from C. Irvine, A. Morgan, A. Crellin, A. Nisbet & I. Beange (2004). Clinical Implications of the Collapsed Cone Planning Algorithm, *Clinical Oncology*, **16**, 2: 148–154, with permission from The Royal College of Radiologists.

Gambling with Physics—the name Monte Carlo is taken from the famous gambling centre on the Mediterranean. Referring to Chapters 2 and 3, and thinking how photons interactions with electrons happen and how electron interactions with other electrons happen, we could follow one photon and roll dice to decide on each interaction that photon has with an electron, and then assign energy loss to the cells in that electrons path. If we get a computer to do this thousands of times for billions of photons and the electrons they liberate, this is a Monte Carlo calculation.

While more appealing to physicists due to the way they model dose on a more microscopic level, they are still subject to some uncertainties due to approximations that are made to keep calculation times reasonably low.

At this time, they are still relatively 'new to the market' but it has been observed that in tissues with roughly the same atomic number but different densities, such as fat, muscle, and lung, Monte Carlo and superposition dose models give similar results, but Monte Carlo delivers more accurate results in soft tissue within and adjacent to bone.

Chapter 10

Imaging for treatment delivery: Image-guided radiotherapy

Frances Lavender

10.1 What is IGRT?

Image-guided radiotherapy (IGRT) uses images taken immediately before or during treatment, to adjust patient setup, track motion, or to create, adjust or select the treatment plan.

10.2 Types of imaging used for IGRT

10.2.1 Planar images (kV or MV)

Most linear accelerators contain an X-ray tube and kV detector panel that are used for imaging at kV energies. Some treatment rooms may contain two X-ray tubes and detectors, positioned at 90 degrees with respect to each other to acquire orthogonal kV images of the patient. Planar kV images are compared to digitally reconstructed radiographs (DRRs) created at planning (see section 8.8). Images can also be acquired at MV energies using the linac source and an MV detector panel.

10.2.1.1 Why do kV images have better contrast than MV?

Let's have a brief review of photon interactions.

As you will remember, there are five main types of interactions of photons with matter (see Chapter 2): Rayleigh or elastic scattering, photoelectric (PE) absorption, Compton scattering, pair production, and photonuclear interactions (section 2.4). At energies of 10 kV to 6 MV, most interactions occur via the PE or Compton effect. The probability of PE absorption increases with decreasing photon energy. Therefore, more PE interactions will occur at kV energies than at MV energies. This results in better contrast in kV images compared to MV images.

As the probability of PE interactions is proportional to the cube of the atomic number of the material (Z^3), kV images have good contrast between materials of different densities (i.e. bone, tissue, air). kV planar imaging is commonly performed for patient setup of treatment sites that will be matched on bony anatomy; for example, supraclavicular fossa (SCF) fields or spine treatments. The kV planar images are compared to the DRR, matched on bony anatomy, and shifts applied to the couch.

MV imaging is however useful for certain applications. Artefacts from high density materials such as metallic implants and dental fillings are significantly less on MV imaging compared to kV imaging. Additionally, MV planar imaging can use radiation from the treatment beam. This means there is no additional dose to the patient from imaging. For example, this may be used during breast treatments with images being reviewed before the next fraction (Figure 10.1).

10.2.2 Cone-beam CT

The most common pre-treatment imaging technique is cone-beam CT (CBCT). The linear accelerator (linac) has a kV source and a detector attached to the gantry as shown in Figure 11.10. The kV source is an X-ray tube that emits a cone-shaped beam

(a)   (b)

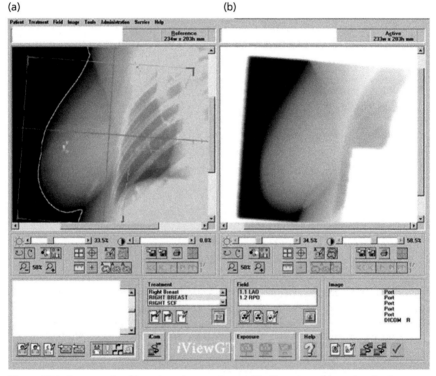

Figure 10.1 An example of how imaging can be used in the setup of breast patients. An MV image (b) is taken immediately before treatment and compared to the digitally reconstructed radiograph (a) (DRR, defined in Chapter 9). Images are acquired from two angles. The system calculates the couch shifts that would be required to match the external breast contour and the chest wall contour on the two sets of images. The treatment radiographer will check the matching and apply the couch shifts. The patient position should now match the planned treatment position. Alternative types of imaging such as CBCT or surface mapping techniques are commonly used to set up breast patients. Images from iView GT imaging, Elekta

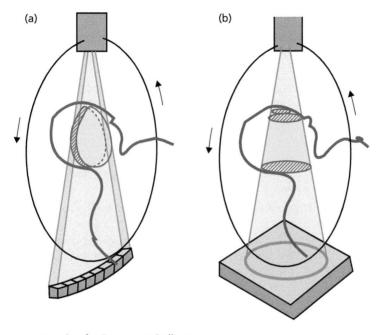

- Imaging for Treatment Delivery

- CBCT

Figure 10.2 Conventional CT scanners use a narrow fan-beam and narrow bank of detectors (a). Consequently, a thin 'slice' of the patient is irradiated with each rotation. CBCT systems on linacs use a cone-beam and flat panel detector so the whole volume of the patient to be imaged is irradiated with a single rotation (b). This results in increased scatter in the final image compared to conventional CT.

of X-rays, as shown in Figure 10.2. These are detected by the kV panel. By rotating the gantry whilst the X-ray beam is on, we acquire a type of computed tomography (CT) scan, known as a CBCT scan. Metal filters called 'bow-tie' or 'half-bow-tie' filters are attached to the X-ray tube to attenuate components of the beam to improve image quality.

A CBCT scan has the following similarities to a diagnostic or planning CT scan:

- **Photon interactions:** As the X-ray beam travels through the patient, some photons undergo interactions with the tissue (e.g. photoelectric or Compton interactions). The X-rays that reach the detector are used to reconstruct a volumetric image.

- **Reconstruction:** Images are reconstructed using filtered back-projection or iterative reconstruction.

- **Artefacts:** Both images are subject to streaking artefacts from high density materials (e.g. metals in prosthesis or dental fillings).

There are also some important differences:

♦ **Dose:** CBCTs are usually lower dose than most diagnostic or planning CTs. The dose depends on the exposure parameters and should be optimized according to its purpose (i.e. for different treatment sites, size of patient, field of view).

♦ **Rotations:** CBCT acquisitions consist of a single rotation (360°) or partial rotation (< 360°) around the patient. In a diagnostic or planning CT scan, the X-ray source can rotate hundreds of times around the patient.

♦ **Geometry:** CT uses a narrow, collimated X-ray beam and a narrow set of detector banks. CBCT uses a cone-shaped beam and a large detector panel. Consequently, in CBCT, radiation scattered through a large range of angles will be incident on the detector resulting in more noise in the image.

♦ **Image quality:** Due to the lower exposure parameters, the acquisition geometry (fan beam with only one rotation around the patient), and the increased scatter in the dataset, CBCT images usually have lower image quality than diagnostic or planning CTs. CBCTs will appear noisier, with poorer soft tissue contrast, and more artefacts.

♦ **CT number:** Although each voxel in a CBCT image has a CT number with units of Hounsfield units (HU), the CT number may not be uniform across the field of vision (FOV). CBCT systems may also not be calibrated to give stable CT numbers.

Other types of CBCT:

♦ **Extended/stitched CBCT:** The sup/inf length of a CBCT is limited by the size of the detector panel. Multiple CBCTs can be acquired consecutively and then 'stitched' together by the imaging software.

♦ **4D-CBCT:** To see organ movement on CBCT data, each image can be assigned or 'binned' to a different section of the respiratory cycle. This is useful, for example, in lung treatment so that the position of the tumour in each phase can be reviewed or the images can be played consecutively in a 'movie' so see the extent of tumour motion and its path. To achieve this, we need to measure the respiratory trace during acquisition of the imaging data. This process is described in the section on 4D CT in Chapter 8. To achieve sufficient image quality, 4D imaging usually results in a higher dose to the patient than 3D imaging.

♦ **Gated CBCT:** This is when images are only acquired during specific parts of the respiratory cycle. For example, we could acquire images during a window around peak inhalation.

♦ **MV-CBCT:** A CBCT scan can also be acquired using the MV panel on a linac and the MV radiation from the target inside the gantry. MV-CBCT is not commonly used clinically due to its poorer soft tissue contrast and increased dose compared to kV-CBCT.

10.2.3 Surface or marker monitoring

Various systems use different techniques to track surface movement or the movement of markers:

Optical surface monitoring: By projecting light from multiple angles onto the patient's skin and detecting the reflected light with multiple cameras, the system can generate a real-time image of the patient surface.

Infrared cameras and reflectors: By attaching a block with reflective markers to the patient's chest and using a camera system to emit and image infrared light, the movement of the reflective markers can be recorded and converted into a respiratory trace.

Electromagnetic sensors and transponders: Transponders are devices that transmit a signal when they receive a specific signal. A 4D electromagnetic sensor array positioned above the patient can be used to track the motion of transponders. These transponders can either be internal (e.g. inserted into the lung or prostate) or surface transponders (attached to the skin).

10.2.4 MRI and ultrasound

Other imaging modalities such as ultrasound and magnetic resonance imaging (MRI) are also used for image guided radiotherapy. A description of how ultrasound and magnetic resonance (MR) images are acquired is given in the imaging for treatment planning chapter (section 8.5). Examples of how MR and ultrasound images are used for adaptive radiotherapy on MR-linacs or in brachytherapy are given in section 10.7.

10.3 Is everything the same as the planning CT?

As discussed in Chapter 8, CT is the most common modality used for planning datasets. During planning, the treatment planning system has been used to calculate the dose distribution to the planning CT. However, the patient and their internal anatomy will not be in the same position at treatment as they are in the planning CT due to inter-fraction and intra-fraction motion. Any differences between the patient position, anatomy, or organs at risk (OAR) shape will result in differences between the calculated and delivered dose distributions. Therefore, imaging is used to:

1) Detect what differences exist

2) Take action to minimize these differences

3) Evaluate the effect of any remaining differences on the dose distribution and decide whether to deliver the treatment

10.4 Setup of patient

The simplest type of image-guided radiotherapy (IGRT) is using imaging to optimize the setup of the patient. A common workflow is to acquire a cone-beam CT image immediately before treatment is delivered. An example workflow is given below.

1) The patient enters the treatment room and lies on the linac couch.

2) The radiographers move the couch to visually align the patient's tattoos (made at the planning CT) to the treatment room lasers. The intersection of the lasers defines the treatment room isocentre.

3) 'Setup instructions' will have been made during planning. These will state the distance between a point defined by the patient's tattoos (e.g. a user origin or localization point) to the treatment plan isocentre. The treatment radiographers move the couch sup/inf, ant/post, left/right by the distances stated in these setup instructions.

   Steps 1–3 have positioned the patient so that the isocentre of the treatment plan should be approximately aligned to the isocentre in the treatment room. Images are taken to check that the target volume is in the desired position. This can then be fine-tuned using small couch shifts.

4) Acquire a CBCT image.

5) The radiographers register or 'match' the CBCT to the planning CT. Depending on the treatment site, the registration or 'matching' will be performed to different anatomical features, for example bone, soft tissue, or fiducials.

6) The imaging software calculates the distances between the CBCT and the planning CT.

7) The couch shifts are applied.

8) Treatment is delivered.

It is important to consider the uncertainties and potential sources for error in this workflow:

10.4.1 Example 1: Rotations

The shifts calculated by the imaging software will not be accurate for all scenarios. For example, if the treatment room has a six degree of freedom (6DoF) couch, then it may be possible to correct for both translations and rotations. However, if the couch can only move in the x, y, z directions, then rotations of the patient cannot be completely corrected for. The software can be asked to calculate translations only, but the operator must be aware that there may be increased uncertainties associated with these translations.

10.4.2 Example 2: Matching using bones or soft tissue

CT and CBCT images have good contrast between materials with significantly different densities, such as bone and soft tissue. Matching using bony anatomy can give a good indication of the global alignment of the patient. However, there may not be rigid geometry between bone and the planning target volume (PTV) or OARs, so an excellent bony anatomy match does not mean that the PTV or OARs are in the desired treatment position. A common error when matching on bony anatomy is to match on the wrong vertebra. Additional planar kV images or a longer CBCT length may be included in a workflow to avoid this. Matching may also be performed on soft tissue. Note that compared to MRI, CT has poor soft tissue contrast and CBCT has even poorer soft tissue contrast, as seen in Figure 10.3.

10.4.3 Example 3: Matching using fiducials

For prostate radiotherapy we may register to fiducials such as gold seeds. These are implanted into the prostate by an interventional radiologist before the patient's planning

(a)   (b)

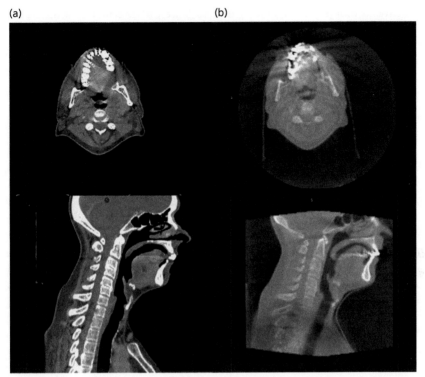

Figure 10.3 Transverse and sagittal Planning CT images (a) and CBCT images (b). The CBCT can be easily identified by its limited field of view and poorer soft tissue contrast compared to the planning CT. Note the streaking artefacts from dental fillings exist in both modality but look slightly different due to the differences in acquisition geometry and reconstruction.

CT. Errors may arise when using fiducial markers because they can migrate. This is minimized by leaving a gap of several days between the implant and the planning CT, during which the fiducial position stabilizes. Also, the geometry of the markers needs to be fit for purpose. If there are three fiducials in different planes of the prostate, these can be used by the software to calculate both rotations and translations. However, if fiducials are aligned in the same plane, or if there are fewer than three fiducials, then rotations cannot be accurately calculated.

10.4.4 **Example 4: Geometry**

For a CBCT acquired by rotation of kV source and detector around the patient, there are limitations to which geometries these can be acquired. For example, if the patient is on a breast board, set to a high angle, or has one arm raised, there may not be enough clearance to acquire a CBCT without the imaging panel colliding with the patient. This may mean that the CBCT is acquired using only a partial rotation around the patient. This is especially useful for acquiring imaging data in these scenarios, but may result in more noise in the image, or in a smaller field of view. Similarly, a treatment field may be delivered with the couch set to 90 degrees. Since CBCTs cannot be acquired with this geometry, the CBCT will need to be acquired with the couch set to zero degrees and then the couch rotated. Care should be taken in this scenario to quantify how much the patient moves when the couch is undergoing such a large rotation.

10.5 Tracking

The meaning of tracking is just as you would expect it to be: the radiation beam follows the movement of the target! Tracking can either be by imaging/measuring the position of the target position, or by monitoring the position of a surrogate whose motion can be correlated with the target motion. Tracking of the treatment beam is commonly performed by adjustment of multileaf collimator (MLC) positions ('MLC tracking') or by adjustment of the linac targeting system, as discussed in the example below.

10.5.1 Example: CyberKnife® lung tracking

The CyberKnife® system (section 11.6.1) has two kV sources attached to the ceiling, and two kV detector panels inserted into the floor to acquire orthogonal planar kV images. For lung treatments, the patient may also be asked to wear a special vest, to which infrared light emitting diodes are attached. As the patient breathes, the movement of these diodes is detected by a camera and converted into a respiratory trace. An advantage of using diodes instead of kV images is that they do not use ionizing radiation and so do not contribute to patient dose. Ideally, we would therefore like to just use the diode trace to 'track' the path of the tumour. However, the diodes are only a surrogate for tumour motion. We need to establish how the diode motion correlates to the tumour motion. This is done by acquiring orthogonal kV images for each part of the respiratory cycle to create a model that correlates tumour position (known from kV images) to the respiratory trace (detected from diode motion). Once the model has been acquired, the frequency of kV image acquisition can be reduced. Newly acquired kV images are then used to 'check' that the model is still valid, without us having to use kV imaging to detect the tumour position for the whole duration of the treatment. The CyberKnife® system uses the model to aim the robot so that the treatment beam tracks the position of the tumour. If the model becomes invalid, for example if the patient coughs or their breathing pattern changes, the system automatically interrupts the treatment beam and a new model will need to be created.

10.6 Gating

Gating can be a useful technique for imaging or treating parts of the body where movement is unavoidable. Gating means that an anatomical movement trace (e.g. respiratory or cardiac) is measured and then used to control the timing of an action. For example, gated imaging can describe the acquisition of images at specific points in the respiratory cycle (e.g. gated CBCT). Gated radiotherapy means that the treatment beam is switched on when, for example, a lung tumour is only in a specific section of the breathing cycle. An advantage of gated radiotherapy is that the internal target volume (ITV) will be smaller compared to non-gated treatments, reducing the dose to healthy tissue.

10.6.1 Example 1: DIBH/VIBH

One example of gating in radiotherapy is breath-hold gating, which is frequently used for breast treatments. For deep inspiration or voluntary inspiration breath-hold (DIBH/VIBH) techniques, the patient is asked to take a deep breath in and hold their breath. The treatment beam is switched on whilst the patient is holding their breath. The breath-hold technique increases the volume of the lungs, therefore increasing the distance between the heart and the tangential breast treatment beams. This can reduce the dose to the heart. The respiratory trace can be measured using a reflective block attached to the patient's chest and an infrared camera system or using surface mapping or imaging. Alternatively, spirometry systems can be used to assist the patient to breathe in a specific volume of air and hold at that level.

10.6.2 Example 2: Gated VMAT

Volumetric modulated arc therapy can also be gated, which can be useful for thoracic or abdominal treatments. The system can either employ either phase-gating or amplitude-gating. In phase-gating, the treatment beam is switched on whenever the patient is in a specified phase of the breathing cycle. In amplitude-gating, the beam is on when specified amplitude is reached, irrespective of where this occurs during the respiratory cycle.

10.7 Adaptive radiotherapy

10.7.1 What is adaptive RT?

Adaptive radiotherapy uses images acquired at the time of treatment to select or modify the treatment plan. This allows a more accurate targeting of dose and consequently reduce the dose to healthy tissue or escalate the dose to the PTV.

Offline planning refers to plans prepared in advance of the treatment session.

Online planning means that the plan is calculated on the day of the treatment session using information acquired during that session (e.g. imaging data).

There are numerous ways of performing adaptive radiotherapy. Three examples are given below.

10.7.2 Example 1: Plan of the day

In this technique, multiple plans are created during the planning stage. For each fraction, the treatment radiographers will acquire a CBCT image of the patient and then select the most appropriate plan based on pre-defined criteria. For example, for external beam RT to the bladder, three plans may be created that have different bladder sizes (small, medium, and large) (Figure 10.4). As the three plans have already been optimized, approved, and checked, there is very little time delay compared to non-adaptive planning, unlike some other types of adaptive RT.

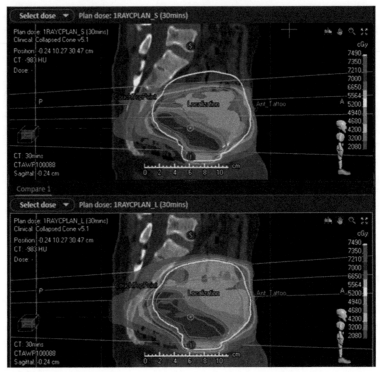

Figure 10.4 Sagittal view of two plans for a plan of the day bladder protocol (taken from Raystation, Raysearch labs). Top plan (for small bladder, low dose PTV (green contour), high dose PTV (blue contour)); Bottom plan (for large bladder, low dose PTV (yellow contour), high dose PTV (red contour)).
Reproduced with permission from RaySearch Laboratories, Stockholm, Sweden

10.7.3 Example 2: Ultrasound for LDR brachy prostate

Low dose rate (LDR) brachytherapy to the prostate using iodine seeds is commonly performed using trans-rectal ultrasound. This allows the clinicians, physicists, and dosimetrists to have real-time images during the procedure. The patient is usually under general anaesthetic and all planning is performed in theatre. An example workflow would be for the brachytherapy needle applicators to be inserted and trans-rectal images acquired. The clinician then contours target and OARs and a physicist or dosimetrist creates a treatment plan. This is reviewed and approved by the clinician. The iodine seeds are then inserted in accordance with the treatment plan. As seeds are inserted, their exact position can be seen on the ultrasound image and the dose distribution calculated. The planned positions of subsequent seed positions can then be adjusted to optimize the treatment plan. This is illustrated in section 12.6.1.3.

10.7.4 **Example 3: MR-linac**

Magnetic resonance linear accelerators (MRL) allow the operator to acquire MR images at the beginning of or during a treatment session (Figure 10.5). Below is an example workflow for a daily adaptive treatment on an MRL.

1) Acquisition of reference CT and MRI

2) Before fraction 1, a treatment plan is created on the reference image, checked, and approved by clinician. Let's call this the reference plan.

3) Patient arrives for fraction 1 and is setup on the MRL couch.

4) MR images acquired. We will call these 'session images'.

5) Session images are registered to the reference image.

6) Session images are contoured. This can be done by using rigid or deformable contour propagation from the reference to session images, followed by manual correction if necessary.

7) The Reference plan may be recalculated on the session image. If dose distribution requires improvement, plan is re-optimized on the session image. In some MRL systems, the plan is re-optimized daily.

8) The online plan is then checked and approved.

9) Whilst the plan is being checked, a verification MR image is acquired.

10) Verification image is registered to the session image.

11) Differences between verification and session images are evaluated to determine whether to proceed with current online plan, apply an isocentre shift to improve patient alignment, or to take alternative actions.

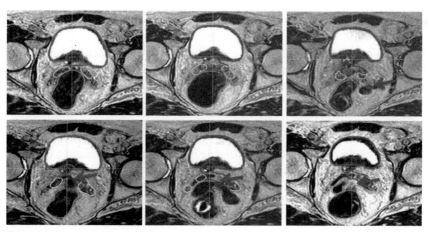

Figure 10.5 Images from six fractions of daily adaptive prostate treatment on an MRL, illustrating the daily positional variability of the OARs and target structures. Contours: CTV prostate (red), CTV SV (lime green), bladder (purple), bowel (green), rectum (orange).

Chapter 11

Beam therapy equipment

Ondrée Severn

11.1 Introduction

The basic principles behind the operation of many of the treatment machines found in a modern radiotherapy department are effectively unchanged since their inception. However, the performance, construction, and control systems employed in equipment used to treat patients today have significantly advanced through modern engineering, technology, electronics, and computers. Adherence to tight mechanical tolerances means that geometric targeting accuracy is improved. Techniques such as intensity modulated radiotherapy (IMRT) and volumetric modulated arc therapy (VMAT) made some untreatable indications now treatable. The introduction of image-guided radiotherapy through integrated imaging technology allows localization and treatment of moving targets. Improved safety and reliability make for an efficient department and improved patient experience.

This chapter will take you through the basic principles of producing a clinical radiotherapy beam and describe the major equipment components required to deliver treatments safely to our patients.

11.2 X-ray production

The production of a clinical X-ray beam whether in the kV or MV range depends on the bremsstrahlung interaction process. This process occurs when a target of made appropriate material is bombarded by an energetic beam of electrons and is discussed earlier in section 2.3.

11.2.1 Target design

The choice of target material is influenced by the fact that bremsstrahlung intensity is proportional to the atomic number Z, that is the number of protons in the nucleus of the material; the higher this number the better. The material needs to be in a manageable form, preferably a solid that is robust and easily machinable in standard engineering processes. Tungsten (a metal with a high Z of 74 and a high melting point of 3422 °C) and tungsten alloys are ideal as they can withstand the extreme heating that occurs during X-ray production.

The type of target is also influenced by the directionality of the X-rays produced. Figure 11.1 indicates how this changes with increasing energy of incident electrons.

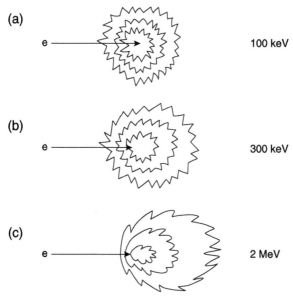

Figure 11.1 a) At superficial energies the bremsstrahlung X-ray production is virtually omni-directional. b) As the energy increases to the order of several 100s of keV there is greater directionality to the X-ray beam. c) For energies in the megavoltage range the X-ray beam is primarily directed forward.

At the low (keV) energy, where X-ray production is isotropic, sufficient X-ray intensity can be obtained with the target turned at an angle to the direction of the electron beam. At the MeV energy level, the greatest intensity comes *through* the target, so we call this a 'transmission target'.

11.2.2 **How are electrons generated for X-ray production?**

As you remember from section 2.3.1, the electrons required to create the clinical X-ray or electron beam are generated by 'thermionic emission'. A metal is heated so that its electrons become very energetic and leave the surface of the metal creating an 'electron cloud'. X-ray machines of all energies use tungsten filaments as the source of electrons for the accelerated electron beam. The intensity of the X-ray beam produced depends on the number of electrons emitted from the filament which in turn is related to the electrical current applied to the filament. This current is controlled electronically to respond to any changes in the mains electrical supply and stabilize the electron beam intensity.

11.3 **Megavoltage linear accelerator (the linac)**

The linac is the workhorse of the modern radiotherapy department, designed by pioneers who developed megavoltage machines in the 1950s. Most are compact machines capable of rotating round the patient and delivering high dose rates, with all

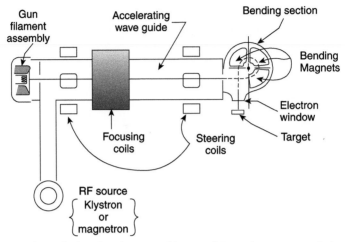

Figure 11.2 Schematic showing the general layout of the major components found in a linear accelerator producing electron and X-ray beams.

with similar general layout and components. Figure 11.2 illustrates the typical layout of the major components of a linac.

The requirements for clinical beam production are:

Electron generation	Electrons must be generated and injected into the waveguide
Electron acceleration	Electrons are accelerated to speeds close to that of light
Beam transport	Electrons are focussed for use as a clinical beam or incident on a target to generate photons through bremsstrahlung
Treatment head	Beam is modified for clinical use

11.3.1 Electron generation, acceleration, and beam transport

11.3.1.1 The gun

The 'gun' filament assembly (section 11.2.2) produces electrons by raising tungsten to a high temperature through electrical heating.

11.3.1.2 The waveguide

The high energies produced in modern medical linacs have been made possible by the controlled use of electromagnetic (EM) radiation. It was found that EM radiation could be propagated along metal conduits called *waveguides*, the wavelength and propagation speed of the EM wave being determined by the dimensions of the waveguide. An essential aspect of the waveguide is that it aligns the electrical component of the EM wave to the direction along which acceleration is required. A charged particle, in our case an electron, can then be accelerated by this electric field.

The electrons are accelerated under the action of EM waves at a frequency of approximately 3 GHz (EM waves of this frequency are called *microwaves*, see Figure 1.7) along the waveguide. There are two types of waveguide: standing wave and travelling wave guides.

In the travelling type, the electrons are carried along on a wave like a surfer, accelerating due to the changes in cavity size so the electron and wave move together. In the standing type, the wave stays still, but the maximum and minimum points of the wave switch place, like a skipping rope. In both cases the electron always sees an accelerating force of a positive (attractive) potential ahead of it and a negative (repulsive) potential behind it.

11.3.1.3 RF wave production

The microwaves are produced in either a klystron or a magnetron. The magnetron, being physically smaller, can fit into the rotating gantry to allow compact design. The klystron, which must be mounted independently of the gantry, can deliver the higher power levels required for high energy linacs. A pulse modulator provides high voltage/current pulses to the microwave generator, timed with supply to the electron gun. This results in the radiation from a medical linear accelerator being pulsed as opposed to continuous.

11.3.1.4 Focusing and steering coils

The repulsive force between the electrons causes the beam to disperse as it travels along the accelerating waveguide. This is countered by using a magnetic force from focusing coils which are wound around the accelerating waveguide and produce a magnetic field parallel to the direction of the electron beam. Coils at the beginning of the waveguide steer the electrons immediately after they are injected and further steering coils at the end of the waveguide correct for deflections due to geomagnetic and other external influences. These are set optimally but require continuous control throughout treatment delivery.

11.3.1.5 Bending the electron beam

The accelerating waveguide can be in line with the treatment axis or perpendicular to it. In the latter case, the path of the electrons needs to be bent through a right angle to hit the target by a series of bending magnets. Designs of bending magnets vary between linac manufacturers. Some use a series of magnets that steer the electrons along a slalom trajectory before the final bend others bend the electron path through a full 270 degrees back onto the target. What both have in common is that they are 'achromatic'; electrons exiting the waveguide with slightly differing energies can be focused onto the same point on the target.

11.3.1.6 Vacuum and cooling systems

The electron gun, accelerating waveguide, and beam transport system must all operate in a vacuum to prevent the scattering of electrons by collision with gas molecules. Interlocks prevent the use of the linac if the pressure in these areas exceeds a predetermined value. Many components within the linac also require cooling via a chilled water supply, which helps prevent overheating and failure.

11.3.2 The treatment head

11.3.2.1 X-ray production

The X-ray beam originates in a transmission target (section 11.2.1) directly in the line of the path of the electron beam immediately after it exits from the accelerating wave-guide and the bending section. The exiting X-ray production is collimated into the raw beam by a conical primary collimator (Figure 11.6); this defines the largest available treatment area.

11.3.2.2 Flattening the treatment beam

The raw beam has peak intensity in the forward direction (Figure 11.3). Conventionally the aim in radiotherapy has been to deliver as uniform a dose as possible to the target, a task made easier before the days of treatment planning computers and intensity modulated delivery, by modifying the raw beam so that it is uniform across the width of the field. The beam is 'flattened' by inserting a flattening filter on a moveable carousel in the path of the beam. These are generally made from steel, shaped like a witch's hat, and provide the max-imum attenuation in the centre of the field. The detailed shape of the filter is specific to the energy of the X-ray beam and the beam profile which it is intended to produce.

11.3.2.3 Flattening filter-free (FFF) mode

Treatment planning techniques such as IMRT and VMAT do not require a flattened beam profile and most linac manufacturers offer the option of treating in flattening filter-free (FFF) mode. Removing the filter results in considerably higher dose rates on the central axis (up to four times that of the flattened beam) which makes it beneficial

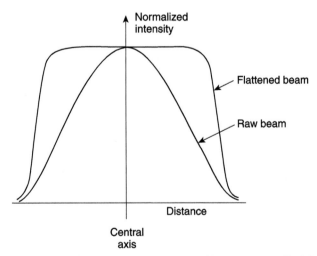

Figure 11.3 Comparison of a raw MV X-ray beam profile, with the profile following the flattening filter.

for treatments delivering a large dose per fraction. It also reduces the head scatter (section 6.3) that is produced from photon interactions with components in the treatment head and therefore the out-of-field leakage radiation from the treatment head. The resulting beam will be of a lower average energy as the beam hardening effect of the filter has been removed and some linac manufacturers have increased the incident energy of the electrons to compensate for this.

11.3.2.4 Monitoring dose and beam parameters

Following flattening of the beam the X-rays pass through two transmission 'monitor' ionization chambers. The ionization chambers control the dose delivered and continuously monitor the beam characteristics. Two chambers (CH1 and CH2) provide redundancy in the system. The first is the primary and provides a signal to terminate the beam after the required dose (defined in monitor units) has been delivered. The second acts as a safety back up and will terminate the beam if the first fails. If both fail, there is also a timer to stop the beam!

The chambers are divided into paired segments that monitor the beam position and energy. These feed signals back to the electron gun and steering coils throughout treatment delivery to constantly maintain dose rate and beam steering and ensure a stable, symmetric beam profile as indicated in Figure 11.4.

11.3.2.5 Shaping the clinical beam

The maximum available treatment beam size must be shaped to match the desired treatment area using a substantial secondary collimation system. This consists of two sets of opposing 'jaws' (secondary collimators) and/or multileaf collimators.

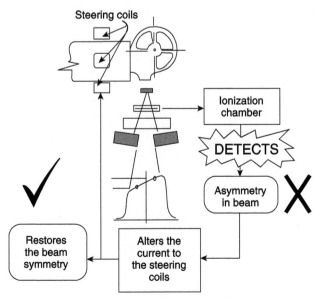

Figure 11.4 The major components involved in automatically steering the electron beam to maintain a uniform and symmetrical X-ray beam.

Secondary collimators—Four thick tungsten or lead alloy blocks paired as X and Y jaws are mounted at the end of the treatment head, one set above the other. The jaws are of a fixed size but can move independently to create a full range of symmetric or asymmetric rectangular field sizes. The collimator assembly can be rotated to alter the orientation of the shape. The edges of the jaws are shaped to match the divergence of the X-ray beam and typically have a transmission of < 0.5%. Moving the jaws across the treatment area during beam delivery can be used to create a wedged profile, this is called a dynamic or virtual wedge (see Chapter 6).

Multileaf collimators (MLC)—Banks of independently moveable tungsten 'leaves' with widths at the isocentre ranging from 2.5 mm to 10 mm are mounted below the jaws. The narrower leaves are usually in machines designed for stereotactic use. They can be moved independently into the field to create complex concave and convex shapes (Figure 11.5). Transmission between the leaves is greater than through them but is reduced by a tongue and groove design. By rapidly changing the beam shape and providing multiple beams within the overall field or by dynamic control of the MLC whilst the machine is irradiating (section 9.10) the intensity of the beam can be modulated; this is IMRT.

11.3.2.6 Accessories

Removable beam modifying devices can be attached to the head of the linac beyond the fixed collimation via an accessory holder. Examples of these are a physical wedge to alter the beam profile, shaped shielding blocks to complement or replace MLC, shaped

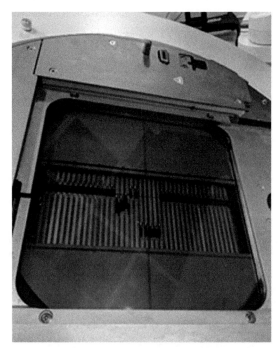

Figure 11.5 Linac treatment head showing shaped field segments formed by multileaf collimators.

attenuating material (compensators) to compensate for patient shape or varying depth of target or, in the case of electrons, an additional external collimator. All are interlocked to ensure that the correct accessory is in place for an individual patient treatment. The use of such accessories is becoming increasingly rare.

11.3.2.7 Clinical electron beam

As well as producing X-rays, linacs are also used to deliver electron treatment beams (Chapter 7). In this mode, the transmission target is automatically moved out of the beam and a thin window allows the accelerated electrons to emerge from the vacuum system. To broaden the narrow electron beam for clinical use, either a scanning technique or some form of scattering material is required.

The predominant technique uses a scattering system, a thin metal foil held on the same carousel as the flattening filters. The foil should be made of a high Z material to increase the scattering but be thin to reduce the X-ray production and contamination of the beam. As the electrons are easily scattered by structures in the treatment head a detachable electron collimator that is brought close to the patient must be used to collimate the beam further (Figure 11.6). These applicators have open sides and

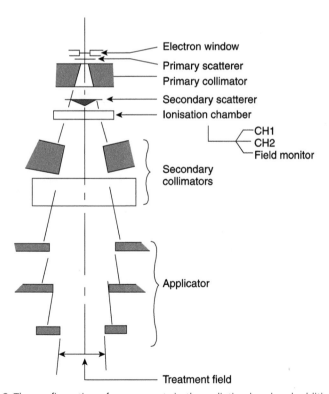

Figure 11.6 The configuration of components in the radiation head and additional collimation devices required when the linear accelerator is used to provide an electron beam.

consist of a set of field trimmers which reduce the field down to the required size. Though they are always rectangular in shape, irregular target areas can be treated by attaching custom built cut-outs made of lead or low-melting point alloy to the end of the collimator.

11.3.3 Calibration of dose output

The absolute output of the machine in Gray (Gy) per monitor unit (MU) is measured following a national protocol or 'code of practice' and this uniformity of approach reduces variability in treatment between institutions. Centres should use an ionization chamber with a calibration that can be traceable to a national standards laboratory (section 5.9). The output of the machine, the dose delivered/set MU, is monitored daily through routine quality assurance (QA) procedures and will ordinarily drift over time making it necessary to periodically re-calibrate the machine. The procedure should be carried out under the supervision of a medical physics expert (MPE) (Chapter 14) and must involve two entirely independent output measurements. The absolute output of the machine in Gy per MU is defined for a standard setup with specified source to calibration distance (SCD), depth of calibration, and field size at a distance of 100 cm from the radiation source. This setup may be different between departments (though most departments employ a set field size of 10 cm × 10 cm, several SCD/depth combinations are in common use) but is fixed within a department. All calculations of treatment plan monitor units stem from this, see section 9.7.

11.3.4 Control systems, dynamic feedback loops, and machine interlocks

Effective and safe treatment delivery relies on several control systems which stop the machine if defined performance parameters are breached. Some control systems are within the accelerator, for example the tuning of the magnetron, the electron emission from the gun, and the steering of the beam. Some ensure the stability of voltage and current supplies. Some form part of a dynamic feedback loop, for example, the detection of field asymmetry by the ionization chamber will generate an electrical signal to alter the current supplied to the steering magnet coils and restore the symmetry of the field. All operate automatically and continually during radiation beam preparation and treatment delivery.

11.3.5 The isocentre

Isocentrically mounted linacs are constructed such that all the main axes of rotation of the gantry, the radiation head, and the patient couch intersect though the same point in space, the *isocentre* (Figure 11.7). In practice the isocentre is bigger than a point; it is a sphere of 1–2 mm diameter. This is because the intersection of radiation axis and gantry rotation shifts slightly with gantry angle due to the weight of treatment head.

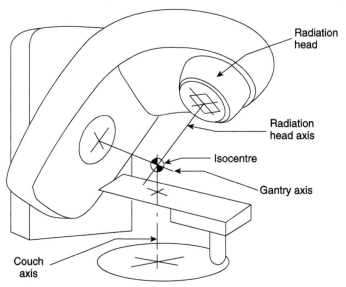

Figure 11.7 The identified axes of a modern accelerator; gantry, radiation head and couch, showing their intersection at the isocentre.

The alignment of the patient such that the centre of the target is at the machine isocentre simplifies treatment with multiple beams. To aid in patient setup and QA procedures, externally mounted room lasers fixed to the walls and ceiling can be adjusted to intersect at the point in space that is the isocentre.

There are two major techniques for which the machines are not used isocentrically: total body irradiation (TBI) and total skin electron (TSE) treatments. For both these types of treatment, the limitation of the accelerator field size is overcome by treating patients further away from the linac, up to 4 m, to achieve full body coverage.

11.3.6 Alignment of patient for treatment, optical indicators, and the treatment couch

11.3.6.1 Optical indicators

The position of the radiation field is visualised using a 'light field' that can be switched on and off using controls on the treatment couch. A bulb and mirror assembly mounted behind the jaws and MLC (Figure 11.8) produces a light field that should be completely coincident with and identical in shape to the radiation field and can be projected onto the patient. A thin window at the end of the treatment head with a cross embedded on it (the 'crosshair' or 'crosswires') is also projected and defines the centre of the radiation field.

A small bulb and scale, the optical distance indicator (ODI) shows the distance of the patient surface from the source of radiation (Figure 11.9). The isocentre is at 100 cm from the radiation source.

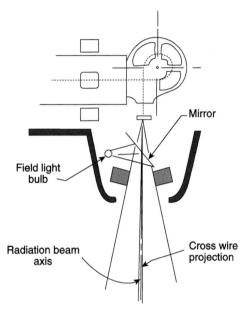

Figure 11.8 The light bulb and mirror assembly create the 'light field' that represents the position of the radiation field.

11.3.6.2 Radiotherapy treatment couch

The linac treatment couch is an integral part of the machine which must perform accurately and reproducibly to provide the most effective treatment. It rotates about the isocentre as shown in Figure 11.7.

Besides isocentric floor rotation the couch has three orthogonal axes of movement allowing the patient to be moved vertically, longitudinally, and laterally for accurate alignment to the radiation beam. Couches are also now available with a further two degrees of rotational motion (in addition to the floor rotation) to correct the patient position for pitch and roll. This reduces the need to physically adjust the patient position on the couch. This is commonly known as a 6D couch, which has three rotations (pitch, roll, and yaw) and three translations (longitudinal, lateral, and vertical).

Couch indexing has become a routine feature of modern couches. Patient alignment devices such as knee rests and head and neck shells lock into the couch in a reproducible way using notches at regular intervals. These locating notches are indexed so that patient setup can be achieved speedily and with a high degree of accuracy on a fraction-to-fraction basis. It is essential that the indexing and supports are the same as on CT and MRI machines to achieve reproducible positioning between treatment planning and delivery.

11.3.7 Integrated image guidance

Reproducible patient positioning and alignment of external markers does not guarantee accurate radiotherapy treatment. Inter- and intra-fractional motion can result

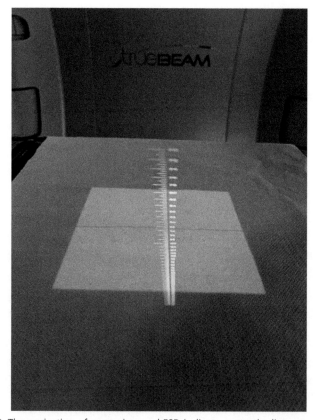

Figure 11.9 The projection of crosswires and FSD indicator onto the linac couch.

in geometric misses or organs at risk (OAR) overdose. However, many of the recent advances in radiotherapy equipment have been in on-treatment imaging and linacs are now equipped with kV and/or MV imaging modalities (Figure 11.10).

11.3.7.1 MV imaging

The MV treatment field itself can be used to provide patient positioning information if the radiation exiting the patient is captured by an electronic portal imaging device (EPID). EPIDs commonly used on radiotherapy linacs are flat panel detectors, accurately positioned in-line with the radiotherapy treatment beam using a moveable arm which is attached to and moves with the gantry. Most are amorphous silicon (aSi) detectors, composed of three main layers. The exit radiation from the patient encounters the first, usually a metal such as copper, and the photons interact with the material to create scattered photons and electrons. The electrons interact with a scintillation material, the second layer, to produce light. The final layer, a panel of aSi photodiodes (one per pixel) convert the light into an electric signal which can be digitised and the resulting image can be compared to digitally reconstructed radiographs (DRRs) produced by the treatment planning system.

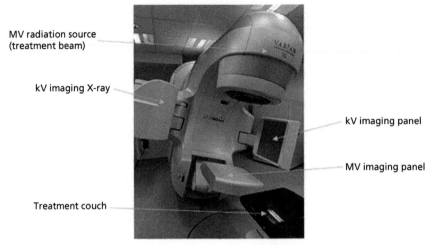

MV radiation source
(treatment beam)

kV imaging X-ray

kV imaging panel

MV imaging panel

Treatment couch

Figure 11.10 A modern linear accelerator equipped with kV and MV imaging capability.

Images can be acquired before treatment with the delivery of a small number of MU, or as fluoroscopic or integrated images acquired during delivery of the radiotherapy treatment.

The contrast in the image is created by the differential attenuation of the incident photons by patient tissue, as in a standard planar diagnostic X-ray. However, the inter-action process that dominates at high (MV) energies is Compton scattering (section 2.4.2). The probability of an interaction occurring via this process is dependent on the electron density of the materials: the relative similarity in electron density of materials found in the human body means that the contrast in MV images is poor compared to those obtained using lower (kV) energy photons.

The functionality of the MV panel and supporting arm should be tested regularly to ensure mechanical safety, stability, and image quality. The panel and positioning arms should be fitted with collision detection to prevent harm to the patient.

However, MV EPIDs can also be used as a tool when performing quality control procedures, for example to image radiation fields to confirm correct jaw calibration, to image MLC shapes to confirm correct field shape, or to record delivered fluences to compare with a treatment planning system for patient plan verifications and *in-vivo* dosimetry, see section 11.3.8.

11.3.7.2 kV imaging

At lower (kV) energies the primary photon interaction process is the photoelectric effect where the probability of interactions is proportional to Z^3. This results in improved contrast between bone and soft tissue and for this reason many radiotherapy linacs are also now fitted with an additional kV source and detector.

The kV source and detector are very similar to a standard diagnostic X-ray tube and digital detector. The X-ray tube produces photons with user-controlled kV (energy) and mA (intensity) settings suitable for a range of patient anatomy and size. It is fitted with filtration to reduce the presence of low energy photons and improve image quality, and blades to collimate the beam to the required field size. They are attached to the linac gantry, again using mechanical moveable arms, at right angles to the treatment beam. Whilst the kV unit rotates with the linac gantry around the imaging isocentre, it will always remain orthogonal to the treatment beam. As all on-line image-matching software acts to move the target to the imaging isocentre, it must be coincident with the radiation isocentre.

For soft tissue targets not adequately represented by bony anatomy or implanted surrogates, the functionality of the kV unit can be extended to produce a kV cone-beam CT (CBCT) (section 10.2.2). The method of acquisition is like that of CT; the linac and therefore the kV unit rotates around the patient, collecting cone-shaped beam projections through the patient from each angle. These are then reconstructed to produce a 3D image. Organs like the bladder and prostate can be better visualised, this allows accurate tumour targeting and introduces the possibility of adaptive treatment.

It is even now possible to acquire a full 4D CBCT image with the patient in the treatment position with data binned according to their position in the breathing cycle and this is especially valuable for tumours near the diaphragm in the lower thorax or upper abdomen.

11.3.8 Transit dosimetry

Whilst the MV planar images suffer from poor contrast between bone and soft tissue they have the benefit of being in-line with the radiotherapy beam and created from the exit radiation from the patient. If the EPID panel is calibrated such that its response can be related to dose, then the captured information can be used to provide valuable information about a patient's treatment delivery (section 15.4.4.2).

Sophisticated software can measure the total fluence collected on the MV panel during treatment delivery, along with the original planning CT or 'on-treat' CBCT, and display this as the delivered dose distribution to the patient. Errors in treatment delivery or patient setup will be highlighted as areas of under- or overdose when compared to the planned distribution.

11.3.9 Gated treatment delivery

Intra-fraction motion, particularly of target volumes that move with breathing, is sometimes accounted for by increasing the margins used at the treatment planning stage. However, many linacs now can 'gate' radiation delivery, that is turn the treatment beam on and off, usually in response to phases in a patient's breathing cycle.

There are several ways to create the gating signal; some systems use a reflective marker block placed on the patient's chest that moves with breathing and can be used to create a breathing trace and others use spirometry to control the radiation. All methods rely on the linac being able to produce a stable dose rate and beam profile almost instantaneously following switching on of the beam.

11.3.10 Record and verify systems

Current radiotherapy treatment deliveries are too complex for plan parameters to be entered manually into the treatment machine console. Instead, record and verify (R&V) systems act both as a database to store patient information and as an interface between imaging systems, treatment planning systems and treatment delivery machines (Chapter 4). The automatic transfer of plan data (e.g. machine settings and prescribed dose) will reduce the risk of treatment errors in radiotherapy, some of which have historically originated in errors from manual entry of treatment parameters.

In most treatments treatment field parameters (including information on required monitor units, beam energy, gantry, collimator and jaw settings, and MLC position and accessories) are transferred directly to the machine from the treatment planning system. Discrepancies between the actual and expected plan parameters will be highlighted and cause a machine interlock preventing the delivery of radiation.

Once the treatment fraction is completed the dose delivered and all on-treatment images are saved back to the database providing a record of treatment and the opportunity for offline review of patient setup. Chapter 4 describes how these different types of data are transferred.

11.4 Kilovoltage X-ray beam machines

The relatively low energy X-rays produced by kilovoltage treatment units mean that they are useful for treating superficial lesions. Units built to provide X-ray beams in the kV energy range are typically mounted on a 'tube stand' attached to the ceiling or floor that can be easy translated or rotated to direct the beam onto the patient (Figure 11.11).

11.4.1 High-voltage circuits

A high-voltage supply is necessary to create a large potential difference, to draw (accelerate) electrons towards the anode. Treatment machines use a feedback system to monitor and respond to changes in supply to ensure a stable voltage is maintained across the X-ray tube.

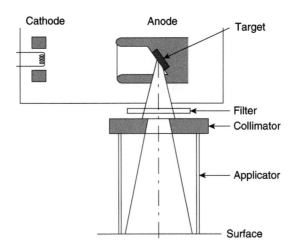

Figure 11.11 Schematic of a kilovoltage (kV) therapy X-ray machine.

11.4.2 Collimation and beam profile

The hooded construction of the anode provides the initial collimation of the beam as the X-rays are generated almost isotropically at the target (Figure 11.1a and b). An aperture then defines the maximum size of conical X-ray beam available, and the final collimation is completed by a removable applicator. Applicators are available in a range of sizes and source-to-surface distances (SSDs) but are usually limited to circular and square apertures and SSDs in the range 20–50 cm. The applicators for use at the lower energy range of the treatment machine have the shorter SSD and are open ended to maximize dose to the patient, those for use at the higher energies have closed ends to compress the patient surface and bring the tumour closer to the source.

The variation of intensity across a kilovoltage beam, referred to as the beam profile, is slightly asymmetric in the cathode/anode direction. This so-called heel effect arises due to absorption of some of the X-rays within the target itself (Figure 11.12). In all directions there will be significant drop off in beam intensity from the central axis of the beam towards the edge and it is important to allow an adequate margin for this when planning a patient's treatment.

11.4.3 Beam energy and filtration

The X-ray beam from any target consists of a continuous spectrum across a range of energies up to the maximum accelerating potential (kVp) with spikes of intensity at energies determined by the target material due to characteristic X-rays (Chapter 2). So for a 120 kV machine, 120 keV will be the accelerated electron energy, the maximum X-ray photon energy will be 120 keV, and the beam can be called 120 kVp. This spectrum of energies is modified using removable filters to remove lower energy X-rays (known as beam hardening) and so reduce the dose to the skin. Each is designed only for use with a particular kV setting and machine interlocks prevent exposure with an incorrect filter in place.

The energy characteristics of the beam are often referred to as the beam 'quality' and depend on both the accelerating potential and the filtration. The beam quality is specified in terms of the half value layer (HVL) which is the thickness of the metal layer

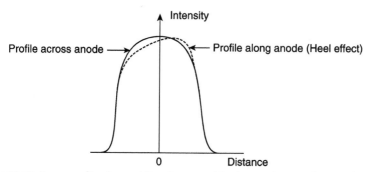

Figure 11.12 Beam profiles from a kilovoltage machine beam along and across the target.

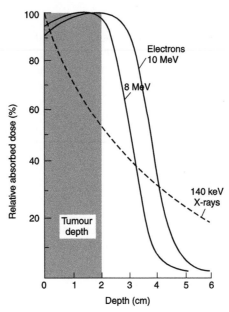

Figure 11.13 Comparison of the percentage depth dose curves from kV X-rays and electron beams.

Reproduced with permission from Klevenhagen S. C. (1985). Physics of electron beam therapy, Fig. 3.1. Bristol: © Adam Hilger Ltd.

required to reduce the intensity of the beam by half (section 2.5.2). The percentage depth dose curve for a kilovoltage beam has a maximum at the surface followed by decreasing dose with depth; a typical curve is shown in Figure 11.13, along with the curves of two different energy electron beams for comparison. For the electron beams, a high dose is maintained across a superficial depth while with the kilovoltage beam the dose rapidly falls away across the same depth. Beyond that superficial depth the electron beam dose decreases rapidly, whereas a substantial dose is delivered beyond that depth by the kilovoltage beam.

11.4.4 Control of output

Either a timer or an ionization chamber (also known as a monitor chamber) is used to control the dose delivered. The timer is normally a countdown device and starts when the treatment is initiated. After the set time has elapsed the voltage and current are switched off and treatment ends.

Most modern units use a monitor chamber through which the beam passes, much like a linac (section 11.3.2.4). It terminates the beam when the required number of monitor units (section 9.7.1) has been reached.

11.4.5 Customized shielding

To treat lesions of non-standard size and irregular shape, lead cut-outs positioned on the patient can be combined with a suitable applicator to shape the treatment field. For lesions on the face and close to the eyes, a lead mask can be made based upon a plaster cast of the patient. For treatments that overlap the eye region insertable commercial lead and tungsten eye shields are available. Lead shielding may be used under the lip to protect gums when the nose or lip are treated. Importantly the shields themselves will contribute to the absorbed dose in the patient due to backscattered electrons produced in the material and it may be possible to cover the shield with wax to absorb these (section 7.8).

11.4.6 Calibration of dose output

The calibration of dose output follows the same principles as that for megavoltage machines (section 11.3.3) in that a clear procedure should be followed that is in line with national guidance and demonstrates direct traceability to a national standards laboratory. The current guidance recommends the calibration of low-energy X-rays (50–160 kVp) be performed in air with the use of a mass energy absorption coefficient ratios to determine the resulting dose to water or tissue at the surface of the patient. Medium-energy X-rays (160–300 kVp) can be calibrated in air or at a depth of 2 cm in water. Practically, the choice to determine the absorbed dose at the surface or at depth in a patient will depend on clinical need.

11.5 Cobalt-60 radioactive source machines

An alternative source of megavoltage radiotherapy treatment beams is gamma radiation produced during the decay of certain radioisotopes (section 1.5.4). The isotope, cobalt-60 (^{60}Co), is produced in nuclear reactors and emits 1.17 and 1.33 MeV gamma rays as it decays. The higher energy photons can treat to greater depth than kilovoltage units and a relatively long half-life of just over five years makes it suitable for use in therapeutic radiotherapy.

The relatively simple design of the cobalt-60 unit comprises encapsulated pellets or discs of ^{60}Co housed in a shielded safe with a shutter mechanism to transport the source into an exposed position. The radiation field is defined by a system of movable collimators and penumbra trimmers. The forward scattering of the electrons produced from the ^{60}Co photon interactions produces a skin-sparing effect with a maximum dose at 0.5 cm depth.

Cobalt units have been superseded by linacs in modern radiotherapy departments. However, they represent a relatively simple method to generate a megavoltage treatment beam and may still have a place when the need for highly skilled maintenance and high costs associated with linacs is prohibitive. An exception to this is the use of cobalt-60 sources in dedicated stereotactic treatment machines.

11.6 Specialist megavoltage treatment systems

11.6.1 Stereotactic machines

Stereotactic ablative radiotherapy (SABR) and stereotactic radiotherapy/surgery (SRT/S) techniques deliver high radiation doses to well-defined small volumes with a high geometric accuracy, usually as single or short fraction courses. Localization may use a stereotactic frame or on-board imaging capabilities with or without tumour surrogates such as implanted fiducials. A standard linac can be used to deliver such a treatment, provided the mechanical integrity of the machine is sufficient to meet the requirement for high targeting accuracy, and these are sometimes fitted with higher resolution MLC leaves. There are also several dedicated stereotactic units on the market.

The Leksell Gamma Knife® (Elekta, Inc.) is one such machine. It consists of a hemispherical treatment head around which there is an array of 192 small cobalt-60 (^{60}Co) sources. The sources are focused onto a small treatment volume, the dimensions of which are determined at the treatment planning stage by a choice of fixed tungsten collimators. The unit is isocentric by design but can deliver highly conformal non-spherical distributions by incorporating multiple isocentres into a single treatment plan. Patients can be accurately located within the treatment cavity using a stereotactic frame fixed to the skull which remains in place for pre-planning imaging and treatment, although frameless stereotaxy with integrated cone-beam CT is now also available on the latest generation of machine.

An alternative is the CyberKnife® (Accuray, Inc.), a compact linac delivering 6 MV FFF X-rays collimated fixed/variable collimators or MLC. It is mounted upon a robotic arm capable of delivering non-isocentric, non-coplanar radiotherapy with high geometric accuracy. The location of the target is determined from two orthogonal kilovoltage images, so the tumour must appear radio-opaque or tracking surrogates such as bony anatomy or implanted markers are used. Patient position is corrected via a treatment couch with six degrees of freedom and frequent imaging and subsequent positional correction continues throughout treatment. The CyberKnife can also create computer models on the day of treatment that relate position of the target to points in the patient's breathing cycle. This way the machine can move the beam to follow tumours that move as a patient breathes.

11.6.2 Dedicated intensity modulated machines

Some treatment units are designed specifically with high throughput IMRT treatments in mind. The most common use linac technology and a ring gantry design based on that of a CT scanner (TomoTherapy® or 'Radixact ®' by Accuray). Integrated imaging systems can produce both a megavoltage fan-beam of photons for treatment or kilovoltage CBCT images which are used to localize the target volume. The fan beam of 6 MV photons is modulated by bank of binary MLCs (meaning that they are either open or closed) and a dynamic jaw. The dose is built up in a helix as the gantry spins and the patient moves through the gantry on the couch. The tomotherapy unit can deliver complex dose distributions to large volumes relatively quickly using this modulated approach. Because the spinning gantry is safely housed inside the casing it can move much faster than an open gantry system seen on conventional C-arm linacs.

11.6.3 Magnetic resonance imaging (MRI)-linac

The MR(I)-linac, combines the imaging quality of an MRI unit with IMRT radiotherapy via an FFF linear accelerator. Magnetic resonance images have superior excellent soft tissue definition over CT or CBCT and deliver no radiation dose. Therefore the MR-linac can accurately track radiotherapy targets without the need for surrogates, and multiple image datasets can be acquired without adding to the dose burden.

To produce the MR(I)-Linac, the manufacturers have had to overcome the technical difficulties that arise from the presence of strong magnetic fields next to traditional components of beam generation and steering found in a conventional linac (see section 11.3.1). Furthermore, all QA equipment and immobilization devices must be MRI compatible.

11.7 **Proton beam accelerators**

Proton therapy (see Chapter 3) can deposit large radiation doses to a tumour whilst sparing normal tissue beyond it. This makes them particularly suitable for the treatment of paediatrics and young adults whose normal tissue is still developing.

11.7.1 **Proton acceleration**

Protons (usually produced by heating and ionizing hydrogen gas) are accelerated to energies in the range 200–250 MeV for clinical use. This can be done using either a cyclotron or synchrotron. Synchrotrons accelerate particles on a circular closed path using varying magnetic and electric fields. They can accelerate particles to a range of energies but are very large (the Large Hadron Collider built by CERN has a circumference of nearly 27 km!). Cyclotrons operate by accelerating particles in an outward spiral, using a constant frequency electric field and steered by a magnetic field. They are more compact so are suitable for installing in a room in a proton therapy facility.

11.7.2 **Beam transport**

Accelerated protons are transported to the treatment room via a 'beam line', operating under a vacuum, and bending magnets act to guide and focus the beam. The main beam line may feed several treatment rooms (Figure 11.14) although the beam can only ever be fed to one room at a time.

11.7.3 **The treatment head ('nozzle')**

Single energy protons will deposit their energy over a narrow depth range so to successfully treat a target it is necessary to combine contributions from beams of different energies to create a 'spread out Bragg peak' (SOBP), as described in Chapter 3. Two main delivery systems are currently available, broad beam (passive scattering) and spot scanning (see section 3.5), with the latter becoming the predominant delivery method.

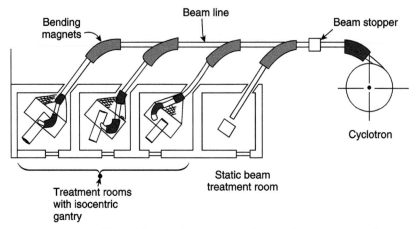

Figure 11.14 A typical layout for a proton treatment facility with a common cyclotron.

11.8 **The machine lifecycle: procurement to decommissioning**

Radiotherapy treatment machines in a busy department will deliver tens of thousands of fractions and it is essential that the procurement process ensures that a new machine meets the needs of the department now and in the future. Any errors in acceptance and commissioning could affect the lives of many patients and so the time taken to obtain accurate, representative data is well spent. (See Figure 11.15).

11.8.1 **Specification and procurement**

- Development of machine specification should take input from all staff groups involved in the delivery of radiotherapy treatments.
- The machine must meet all statutory and regulatory requirements as well as local clinical needs.
- The correct choice of treatment machine may rely not only on modalities and features available but on the ability to beam match and transfer patients between other linacs in the department.

11.8.2 **Installation and acceptance**

- Following the installation, the manufacturer and customer complete a formal customer acceptance protocol (CAP).
- This should include a full demonstration of the capabilities of the machine including geometric and dosimetric performance.
- A critical exam, performed by the manufacturer in conjunction with a radiation protection advisor (RPA), is required by law.

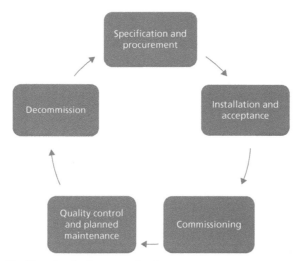

Figure 11.15 The lifecycle of a linear accelerator.

♦ This tests the correct operation of all safety features and warning devices and should include a radiation survey to ensure the safety of operators and patients.

11.8.3 Commissioning

♦ Commissioning is where an extensive set of measurements are undertaken to fully characterize the performance of the machine for clinical use. The critical nature and volume of data required means that this may take a number of months.

♦ These include all the data and verification measurements for dose prediction in treatment planning systems, for example percentage depth doses, profiles, output factors, and wedge factors.

♦ If the machine has been 'matched' to an existing machine, these measurements can be simplified to a comparison with the existing data.

♦ Data collected during commissioning will be used to deliver accurate treatments throughout the lifetime of the machine.

11.8.4 Quality control and planned maintenance

♦ Performance of the machine throughout its lifetime is maintained through planned maintenance and monitored with a quality control programme.

♦ Quality control is also required following repairs to the machine in order to ensure performance has been restored.

♦ Patient-specific quality control may be required to verify the performance of the linac during intensity modulated treatment deliveries (Chapter 9).

11.8.5 Business case for replacement machine and decommission

- Ageing machines will experience increasing downtime due to parts failure and more frequent maintenance requirements.
- Technological advances may render older machines obsolete.
- Both of these will impact on the ability to deliver high quality radiotherapy treatments.
- A business case for a replacement machine must balance these factors against the cost and inconvenience to a busy department of replacing a machine.

Chapter 12

Brachytherapy

Gemma Whitelaw and Susan Corcoran

12.1 Introduction

Shortly after radioactive elements were discovered by Henri Becquerel in 1896, their use as a treatment for cancers and other conditions was established. Dose is delivered by placing the radioactive source in or near the tumour; brachytherapy means 'near treatment', from the Greek word for 'short'. Despite the long history, brachytherapy techniques achieve a high dose close to the source with a rapid dose fall off following the inverse square law (section 2.7). Compared to external beam radiotherapy, this can offer a distinct advantage, with high doses to the target and considerably less to normal tissues and organs at risk; this also means dose can be delivered in large fractions. An additional advantage is that margins to account for set up inaccuracies and organ motion are not required. Brachytherapy is used in a variety of ways in the modern clinic, different sources, placement methods, and treatment areas facilitate a broad and interesting modality.

Historically, radioactive sources were placed manually resulting in potentially hazardous doses to the staff during source placement and throughout the care of the patient with the source *in situ*. To avoid this risk, it became more common to site an applicator or catheter before introducing the source, initially by hand and then by machine. Radioactive sources are categorized according to the rate at which they can deliver dose—either low, medium, or high. Low dose rate (LDR) is when the dose to the tumour is less than 2 Gy per hour, medium (MDR) is 2–12 Gy per hour, and high dose rate (HDR) is greater than 12 Gy per hour.

HDR sources are typically placed using an afterloading device (section 12.3.4) whereas those sources of a lower dose rate may be introduced manually following appropriate radiation protection procedures.

12.1.1 Clinical use

A brachytherapy source can be placed directly into or near a tumour using a variety of techniques. Intracavitary implants are placed into an anatomical cavity adjacent to the target tumour. An example is in the treatment of cervix cancer where applicators are placed in the vagina and uterine canal, and the sources inserted into the applicator. Another example is endobronchial brachytherapy where the source is placed in the bronchus to treat a lung cancer. Interstitial implant techniques are where the radioactive sources are placed directly into the tumour itself, for example in the treatment of prostate cancer using radioactive iodine seeds. Other types are surface applicator methods, for example in the treatment of skin and eye lesions, and intravascular brachytherapy to treat atherosclerotic vascular lesions.

12.2 **Radioactive sources**

Isotopes that are unstable and spontaneously decay to a more stable state are termed radioactive sources (Chapter 1). Sources used for brachytherapy are *sealed* sources; this means that they are solid and encapsulated such that when removed they leave no trace of radioactive contamination. They are encapsulated in an inert metal which may also serve to shield some of the lower energy, less beneficial radiation.

Radium, which was discovered by Marie Curie in 1898, was used as the first brachytherapy source. Although effective, it has disadvantages. Nowadays a range of sources are used for different applications.

12.2.1 **Source requirements**

The requirements of a modern brachytherapy source are varied and depend on its application, however broadly the following criteria should be applied.

- The half life
  - A long half-life allows a source to be used and reused, however methods and costs of disposal must be evaluated and factored into the whole life cost.
  - A short half-life of days to weeks may be more appropriate for brachytherapy where the source is permanently implanted.
  - A very short half-life, in the order of days or less, is generally unsuitable for brachytherapy.
- Type and energy of emission
  - Gamma emission should have an energy high enough to avoid preferential absorption in bone by the photoelectric effect (section 2.4.1) and high enough to minimize scatter, but not so high that it poses radiation protection problems.
  - A beta emitter may be used when the required depth of treatment is very superficial.
  - Otherwise, charged particle emission must be absent or screened.
- Specific activity
  - This is the activity per mass of the source and should be high enough such that the source can both be small enough for implantation and active enough for effective dose delivery.
- Cost
  - Sources can be naturally occurring or manufactured; in both instances the cost of production and distribution should be suitably low. Most modern brachytherapy sources are manufactured.
  - Sources that are not permanently implanted should also have their disposal cost factored in.

- ◆ Decay products
  - Should be non-gaseous and stable.
- ◆ Chemical and physical properties
  - They should have high tensile strength.
  - They should have a high melting point and be able to be sterilized.
  - They should be non-toxic and chemically inert.
  - They should be malleable and easy to manipulate into the desired form.

12.2.2 Commonly used sources

Commonly used sources are described in the Table 12.1, where $_{-1}^{0}e$ denotes an electron.

12.3 Delivery methods

Delivery of brachytherapy has evolved to reduce staff radiation doses and deliver more targeted treatments. Originally, radioactive sources were applied or implanted by hand.

12.3.1 Direct application—historical

12.3.1.1 Gynaecological manual loading

Radium-226, encapsulated into tubes, was inserted by hand into the uterine canal and top of the vagina and used to treat cervical tumours since the 1920s. The Manchester dosimetry system was developed to plan such treatments. With a hazardous alpha emission and a gaseous, radioactive daughter product (radon-222), it was superseded in the 1970s by caesium-137 tubes. Caesium-137 posed less of a radiation protection issue, with a lower photon energy and no alpha emission. An intrauterine applicator and two vaginal applicators (ovoids) were loaded with caesium then inserted into the patient by hand. With a typical low dose rate of 0.55 Gy h^{-1}, treatment times were over several days.

12.3.1.2 Head and neck hairpin interstitial implants

Iridium-192, encapsulated into wire, was inserted by hand into small oral tumours to deliver low dose rate treatments, up until the early 2000s in the United Kingdom. In the form of 'hairpins', it was implanted through surgically inserted metal guides which were then removed, leaving the iridium hairpins *in situ* for several days. A dose of the order of 10 Gy per day was delivered before removal.

Both these techniques resulted in significant staff doses, through insertion, nursing care during treatment, and removal. They are now largely obsolete, thanks to the development of afterloading equipment.

12.3.2 Direct application—current

12.3.2.1 Ocular plaques (surface application)

Radioactive strontium-90 plaques are applied by hand to treat superficial ocular tumours. They take the form of a concave disc with a long handle to maintain distance

Table 12.1 Commonly used brachytherapy sources

Source	Common use	Decay process	Emissions	Half life
Radium-226	Historically for the first brachytherapy treatments, no longer used.	Alpha decay $^{226}_{88}Ra \rightarrow ^{222}_{86}Rn + ^{4}_{2}\alpha + \gamma$	2.45MeV (max)	1600 years
Iridium-192	High dose rate brachytherapy in an afterloader. Also historically as a wire or hairpin.	Beta minus decay $^{192}_{77}Ir \rightarrow ^{192}_{78}Pt + ^{0}_{-1}e + \gamma$	Gamma spectrum, mean 0.38 MeV	73.8 days
Iodine-125	Seeds used for permanent implants, such as prostate brachytherapy.	Electron capture decay $^{125}_{53}I + ^{0}_{-1}e \rightarrow ^{125}_{52}Te + \gamma$	35.5keV gamma photon plus characteristic X-rays at 27.4 and 31.3 keV	59.4 days
Palladium-103	Seeds used for permanent implants, such as prostate brachytherapy.	Electron capture decay $^{103}_{46}Pd + ^{0}_{-1}e \rightarrow ^{103}_{45}Rh + \gamma$	Gamma spectrum, mean 21 keV	17.0 days
Caesium-137	Used in low dose rate remote afterloading units, no longer available in the UK.	Beta minus decay $^{137}_{55}Cs \rightarrow ^{137}_{56}Cs + ^{0}_{-1}e + \gamma$	Gamma, 0.662 MeV	30.17 years
Cobalt-60	High dose rate brachytherapy in an afterloader.	Beta minus decay $^{60}_{27}Co \rightarrow ^{60}_{28}Ni + ^{0}_{-1}e + 2\gamma$	Gamma, 1.33 and 1.17 MeV	5.26 years
Strontium-90	Eye plaques for low penetration surface doses for treatments of ocular tumours.	Beta minus decay $^{90}_{38}Sr \rightarrow ^{90}_{39}Y + ^{0}_{-1}e$ Then $^{90}_{39}Y \rightarrow ^{90}_{40}Zr + ^{0}_{-1}e$	Beta 546 keV, then daughter decays to beta 2.27 MeV	28.7 years effective
Ruthenium-106	Eye plaques used for treatments of ocular tumours.	Beta minus decay $^{106}_{44}Ru \rightarrow ^{106}_{45}Rh + ^{0}_{-1}e$	Beta, 3.54 MeV	374 days

between the source and user. The applicator is applied to the lesion on the eye, using gentle pressure, in an outpatient facility. Treatment planning is simple: a decay calculation of the surface dose rate is used to determine the treatment time, which is usually a few minutes due to the high surface dose rate. Treatments for ocular melanomas are typically fractionated over five days. Applicators may be used for many years, due to the long half-life of strontium-90.

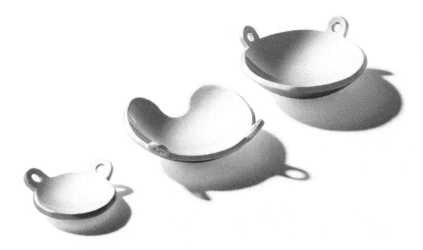

Figure 12.1 Ruthenium-106 ocular plaque.
Reproduced from www.bebig.com with permission from Eckert & Ziegler BEBIG GmbH, Berlin, Germany

Ruthenium-106 plaques (Figure 12.1) are used for deeper ocular tumours up to 6 mm. Also a concave disc, the plaque has suture holes to allow it to be fixed in place for several days as the dose rate is low. Patients need to be cared for as in-patients in single rooms, by nursing staff who have undergone specific radiation training. The plaque is inserted under general anaesthesia and requires sterilization and the use of a specialist microscope. Treatment planning involves the decay calculation of the dose rate at the treatment depth, requiring depth dose tables for each plaque size. New plaques must be purchased every year due to the short half-life of ruthenium-106.

12.3.3 Manual afterloading

Manual afterloading of brachytherapy sources refers to when something that can hold the radioactive source are placed in the patient first—the applicator followed by the placement, by hand, of the radioactive source into that applicator. The source placement is usually after imaging and treatment planning has taken place. This reduces staff radiation exposure.

12.3.3.1 Manual afterloading—historical

12.3.3.1.1 **Interstitial iridium wire implants** In addition to hairpins, iridium-192 was also available in 50 cm wire coils and used in low dose rate brachytherapy in the head and neck.

A flexible tube technique involved surgical insertion of plastic tubes through the treatment site, in an arrangement following a dosimetry system, for example Paris (see section 12.5.1).

Radiographs are taken to determine the iridium wire lengths required. The required wire lengths are cut from the wire coil and inserted into inner tubing. This active inner tubing is then inserted into the outer tubing and clips used to secure the active wire tubing in place. All manipulations of the active wire are performed using long tweezers and forceps, and mobile lead shields are arranged around the patient to protect staff. Patients must be cared for in a single room over the several days of treatment.

Imaging may be repeated to confirm wire positions, and treatment time is calculated using the Paris dosimetry system.

Iridium wire and hairpins are no longer available in the United Kingdom, but similar treatments may be achieved using high dose rate remote afterloaders.

12.3.3.2 Manual afterloading—current

12.3.3.2.1 **Permanent prostate seed interstitial LDR brachytherapy** Low-risk, organ-confined prostate cancer can be treated via the permanent implantation of iodine-125 or palladium-103 encapsulated as seeds, which deliver the prescribed dose over several half-lives. This technique may also be used as a boost following pelvic radiotherapy for intermediate to high-risk tumours.

In the United Kingdom, centres typically use low-activity iodine-125 seeds (see Figure 12.2). The low-energy gamma radiation emitted results in simple shielding requirements: seeds are be transported in small, shielded containers and patients can be discharged home on the same day as the procedure.

Seeds are provided either in cartridges (loose-seed technique) or sutured together in a fixed loading pattern (stranded-seed technique). A combination of the two techniques may also be used.

Centres may use either a one- or two-stage technique:

◆ Two-stage technique: the implant is preceded by a volume study using ultrasound, in the implant position under anaesthesia, to determine the quantity of loose seeds and/or stranded seed loading patterns required, and to produce an intended treatment plan.

◆ One-stage technique: the seed order is determined by a recent transrectal ultrasound (TRUS) or MRI measurement, therefore the patient undergoes one procedure only. The treatment plan is produced dynamically during this single procedure.

The seed implantation and planning technique will vary slightly between centres but for the one-stage technique it is largely as follows:

Setup

◆ The patient is placed in lithotomy position, under sedation or general anaesthesia (see Figure 12.3).

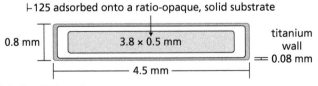

I-125 adsorbed onto a ratio-opaque, solid substrate

0.8 mm | 3.8 × 0.5 mm | titanium wall 0.08 mm
4.5 mm

Figure 12.2 Iodine-125 seed.
Reproduced courtesy and © Becton, Dickinson and Company (BD Bard, crbard.com)

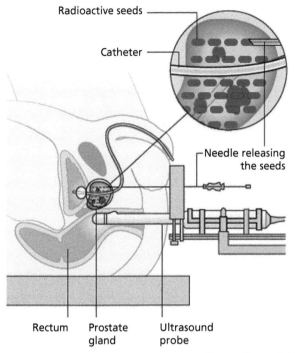

Radioactive seeds

Catheter

Needle releasing
the seeds

Rectum   Prostate   Ultrasound
          gland   probe

Figure 12.3 Prostate brachytherapy needle insertion via transrectal ultrasound- Cancer Research UK image depicting seed insertion.

- A TRUS probe, housed within a stepping unit able to advance and retract to deliver live ultrasound images and positioning information to the treatment planning system, is introduced into the patient's rectum.
- A coordinate template (or 'grid') is attached to the stepping unit and positioned against the perineum, through which several (typically 15–25) fine-gauge metal needles are inserted into the prostate, using TRUS imaging for guidance.

Treatment planning

- The live images of the prostate are directly relayed into the treatment planning system laptop computer, enabling the coordinates of each needle to be recorded into the treatment plan.
- Transverse ultrasound images are captured by the treatment planning system, every few millimetres, by stepping the TRUS probe from the base to the apex of the prostate.
- The prostate and organs at risk are contoured.
- The distribution of iodine seeds within the inserted needles (treatment plan) is planned via volume optimization (see section 12.6.1.3), following the Groupe

Européen de Curiethérapie and the European Society for Radiotherapy & Oncology (GEC ESTRO) recommendations, 2007

Seed implantation

◆ The cartridge of seeds is inserted via a bespoke applicator (e.g. Mick® applicator) which allows the seeds to be pushed through the empty needles and into the prostate in the positions determined by the treatment plan, under ultrasound guidance.

◆ The treatment plan dose distribution is dynamically updated as the implant progresses by the user recording the actual seed positions as viewed on the live TRUS image.

◆ Implantation of stranded seeds is usually carried out via inserting pre-loaded needles, following the treatment plan.

◆ For both loose and stranded seeds, each needle is removed once the seeds have been deposited in the required position.

◆ Additional loose seeds may be planned and implanted to improve the dose coverage.

During and following the completion of the seed implant, radiation monitoring of the equipment and environment must be performed to ensure that no iodine seeds have been misplaced or damaged.

12.3.4 Remote afterloading

Remote afterloading units mechanically introduce the brachytherapy sources into the implanted/inserted applicators in a shielded treatment room. Thus, staff doses are eliminated entirely.

The sources may be positioned to mimic classical brachytherapy and dosimetry systems or optimized to cover target volumes.

12.3.4.1 LDR/MDR remote afterloading—historical

Low dose rate and medium dose rate gynaecological intracavitary brachytherapy was possible using pellet source systems. Source trains in the afterloader unit were programmed as a combination of active (caesium-137) and (inactive) spacer pellets. These would be pneumatically transferred into intrauterine and/or vaginal applicators for a predetermined treatment time (via a treatment planning system (TPS)). Patients would be treated in shielded rooms, with interruptions for nursing care, over 10–24 hours.

This system was not suitable for interstitial treatments due to the relatively large source size (2.5 mm diameter pellets).

12.3.4.2 HDR remote afterloading—current

High dose rate afterloaders use a stepping source and are used widely in UK brachytherapy centres. This is usually an iridium-192 source, less than 1 mm in diameter due to high specific activity, allowing it to fit in intracavitary applicators, and interstitial and intraluminal catheters. The high dose rate means treatments are fractionated for radiobiological reasons, but each treatment time last a few minutes. Iridium-192 has a half-life of 73.83 days so is replaced every three months to make sure treatment times do not become impractically long.

HDR afterloader system features

- Multiple channels to provide multiple applicator/catheter treatment (e.g. prostate brachytherapy)
- A variety of applicators and needles/catheters available (suitable for different treatment sites) to deliver the source into the patient
- Applicators often include material to push sensitive tissues away from very high dose regions close to the HDR source, and to secure the position of the applicator within the body cavity
- Thin flexible source to travel tight curves in applicators
- Programmable treatment console and direct plan transfer from planning system to afterloader system

HDR afterloader operation

- Applicators/catheters connected to afterloader channels by transfer tubes
- A motor/cable system moves the single stepping source through the transfer tubes into each applicator/catheter to a series of programmed positions within the applicator or catheter ('dwell positions')
- The source dwells at each dwell position for varying amounts of time ('dwell times') determined by the treatment plan, to deliver the required dose distribution

HDR afterloader safety features

- Source housed in shielded safe in afterloader, welded to a drive cable
- Back-up secondary timer system
- An automatic check of the transfer tube-applicator/catheter system before the source is exposed using dummy (non-active) source cable
- Built-in source position(s) checks
- Operating system to check that the sources have returned properly
- Back-up power supply
- Manual source return in the event of complete power failure
- Automatic retention of treatment data and history in the event of power failure
- Alarm and status code system to alert user to faults

12.3.4.3 HDR gynaecological intracavitary brachytherapy

Applicators used in gynaecological brachytherapy are made from CT and MRI compatible material, either metal (e.g. titanium) or plastic. They usually are fitted with a plastic cap or segment of different sizes for positioning and dose sparing (section 12.3.4.2).

Vaginal applicators

- Vaginal cylinders for treatment of endometrial and vaginal cancers
- Single central applicator, combined with varying diameter cylinder segments
- Mimic a line source by stepping and dwelling over several centimetres

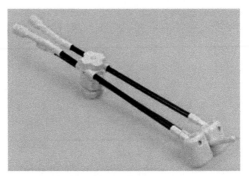

Figure 12.4 Intrauterine tube and ovoids applicator.
Image reproduced courtesy of Elekta (Elekta.com)

- CT or mobile X-ray imaging is used for treatment planning and applicator position verification, either prior to or during the treatment session
- Standard treatments may be delivered via a library of standard treatment plans (section 12.6.1.2)

Intrauterine applicators

- For treatment of cervical cancers
- Intrauterine tube (to deliver the source through the cervix and into the uterus) plus a pair of vaginal applicators ending with plastic ovoids (Figure 12.4) or one ring applicator with plastic cap (to deliver the source into the vaginal fornices). Ring source dwell positions can mimic the ovoid source dwell positions by selecting dwell positions on the lateral sides of the ring or they may be planned in a bespoke pattern
- The ovoids or ring may also be replaced with a vaginal cylinder, providing a single applicator, to treat further into the vagina
- Rectal retractor may be attached to the applicator or packing material inserted into the vagina to reduce rectal dose
- Ovoids and ring caps may have holes so that interstitial needles for improved coverage of large or asymmetric tumours can be used
- CT and/or MR imaging is used for treatment planning and applicator position verification, post-operatively, with treatment delivered a few hours later (see section 12.5.2)

12.3.4.4 HDR interstitial prostate brachytherapy

Fine-gauge metal needles or plastic catheters are inserted under TRUS guidance in a similar set-up to permanent prostate seed brachytherapy (described in section 12.3.3.2). Treatments may be a monotherapy or as a boost to external beam radiotherapy and may be fractionated or single fraction.

- Treatment planning may use either TRUS or CT imaging

- TRUS-based treatment planning allows for intraoperative planning and treatment (as in section 12.3.3.2)
- CT-based treatment planning takes place postoperatively with treatment a few hours later
- Specialized treatment planning systems calculate required dwell positions and times for the HDR source via volume optimization (section 12.6.1.3), following the GEC ESTRO recommendations 2005 and 2013
- Repeat CT-imaging may be used for CT-planned treatments to ensure no catheter movement prior to treatment

12.3.4.5 Other HDR remote afterloading applications

A brief explanation of other less commonly practised HDR brachytherapy techniques follows. Unless otherwise stated, volume or line (at a distance) optimization via CT-planning is used (section 12.6.1).

12.3.4.5.1 **HDR interstitial perineal implants** HDR brachytherapy may be delivered to the anal canal, vagina or vulva via interstitial catheters as part of a bespoke applicator:

- Perineal template comprises of evenly spaced holes to support multiple interstitial catheters
- Optional rigid spacer to displace the rectal or vaginal wall to provide dose sparing where required

12.3.4.5.2 **HDR intracavitary rectum brachytherapy** HDR brachytherapy may be delivered to the rectum, often prior to surgery, via intracavitary applicators:

- Similar to intracavitary vaginal cylinder applicators
- Single or multiple source channels for differential source loading around the cylinder circumference
- May include an incorporated inflatable balloon to improve conformance of the applicator to patient tissues

12.3.4.5.3 **HDR intraluminal bronchus and oesophagus** HDR brachytherapy may be delivered to small bronchial and oesophageal tumours via intraluminal catheters:

- Fine, flexible catheters inserted via the nasal cavity
- Through bronchoscope or nasogastric tube
- Catheters may be inflatable to aid with centring within the lumen

12.3.4.5.4 **HDR skin (surface) brachytherapy** HDR brachytherapy may be delivered to skin cancers, as an alternative to surgery or superficial radiotherapy, using a variety of applicators:

- Tungsten-shielded single-channel surface applicators (with or without a dose-flattening filter) for small skin cancers
- Mesh-style multiple-channel surface moulds ('flaps') to treat large, curved surfaces
- Bespoke 3D-printed surface moulds combined with flexible catheters are now possible

12.3.4.5.5 **HDR head and neck brachytherapy** HDR brachytherapy to the head and neck region may be delivered using intracavitary or interstitial applicators:

- ◆ Nasopharynx mould applicators are designed to fit into the nasopharyngeal cavity
- ◆ Double template and interstitial catheter systems (e.g. noses, tongues)

12.3.4.6 Pulsed dose rate (PDR) remote afterloading—current

Pulsed dose rate afterloaders are like HDR afterloaders but have different software to deliver pulsed treatments, at intervals, to mimic low dose rate intracavitary gynaecological brachytherapy. A lower activity source is required to avoid short dwell times.

12.4 Source specification

It is important that the strength of the source be accurately quantified as this determines the dose of radiation given to the tumour and is programmed into the brachytherapy TPS. Source strength can be defined in a variety of ways, as explored below. In all cases the source strength is determined in a manner that is traceable to a national standards laboratory. This process is termed calibration.

12.4.1 Activity and output

Historically source strength was measured in radium mass equivalent, but now more relevant specifications are used. The concept of activity was explored in section 1.5.5. While activity pertains to the disintegration of a source, for clinical applications we need to consider what is actually emitted from the source so we know what dose the tissue will receive: this is the output. The output is affected by parameters such as the attenuating properties within the source, the filtration of the encapsulating material, source geometry, and a quantity known as the exposure rate constant.

12.4.2 Kinetic energy released per unit mass (kerma) and reference air kerma rate (RAKR)

The kinetic energy released per unit mass kerma) was introduced by the International Commission on Radiation Units (ICRU).

In the modern clinic, sources are commonly specified in terms of the reference air kerma rate (RAKR) which is defined as the kerma rate to air, in vacuo at a reference point at 1 m. Units are $\mu Gy\ m^2\ h^{-1}$.

RAKR is a useful concept because it is directly related to the activity of the source, it is easily converted to dose, it allows for the standardization of units, it is independent of the measurement method and it is the specification used by the national standards laboratory in the United Kingdom—the National Physical Laboratory (NPL). For line sources, RAKR per unit length may be used. More detail is given in the Appendix to this chapter for the keen reader.

12.5 **Dosimetry systems**

Once a brachytherapy source is selected for a particular tumour, the sources then need to be arranged to ensure a standardized dose delivery so that the treatment time can be calculated. The way that this was traditionally performed was to follow a particular dosimetry system.

12.5.1 **Paris system**

The Paris system was, until recently, very commonly used and is still used as a basis for interstitial treatments today. The Paris system works for both the direct placement of sources or for the placement of catheters into which sources are inserted via an afterloader.

12.5.1.1 Paris system rules

Source wires and catheters are placed next to, or through, the tumour according to the following rules:

- They are straight
- They are parallel
- They are of equal length
- They are equally separated
- They should have equal linear activity
- They should be arranged in either a single plane, or a triangular or square formation

12.5.1.2 Paris system calculation

The dose delivered is calculated as follows:

- The basal dose points should be identified. These are on the central plane (perpendicular to and half-way along the sources) and at the mid-points between the centre of two adjacent wires in a planar arrangement, or the centroids of the squares or triangles in a three-dimensional implant. The basal dose points are points of minimum dose on the central plane (see Figure 12.5). The dose rate should be calculated at each basal dose point (to account for decay the dose rate is usually taken from the temporal midpoint of the treatment).
- Calculate the arithmetic mean of the basal dose points.
- Paris system data books contain tables of dose rate to basal dose points for a nominal strength of wire in different geometries, these are called cross-line or escargot curves.
- Calculate the reference dose rate. This is 85% of the mean basal dose rate and is selected because it provides a compromise between dose gradient and volume coverage.
- The reference dose rate can then be used to calculate the treatment time.
- The treatment volume is defined as the area encompassed by the 85% isodose.

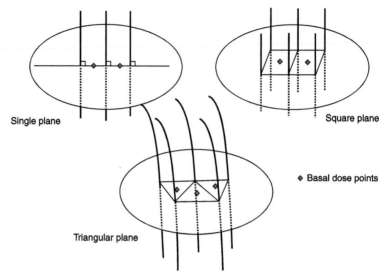

Figure 12.5 Paris system implants.
Reproduced with permission from Hoskin and Coyle, Radiotherapy in Practice: Brachytherapy, Second Edition, 2011, p. 31, Oxford University Press

---

Example calculation: Determine the treatment time

See Figure 12.6

For a single-plane iridium wire implant there are three wires, 40 mm long, separation 10 mm

Prescribed dose = 60 Gy

Source strength of the wire strength at mid-implant = 0.5 μGyh^{-1}mm^{-1} at 1 m

Cross-line curves for nominal source strength (AKR): 1.0 μGyh^{-1}mm^{-1} at 1 m

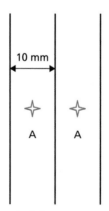

Figure 12.6 Example Paris system calculation.

1) Calculate **distance** from each basal dose point (A) to each wire:

   2 wires @ 5 mm

   1 wire @ 15 mm

2) Look up the **basal dose rate** (BDR) for each point from each wire.

   Use cross-line zero curve—the midplane through the wires:

   2 wires @ 5 mm = 0.6 Gy h^{-1} × 2
   1 wire @ 15 mm = 0.1 Gy h^{-1}
   Total BDR @ point A = 0.6 × 2 + 0.1 = 1.3 Gy h^{-1}

3) **Calculate the mean BDR:**

   1.3 Gy h^{-1} (it is the same for each point in this case)

4) Correct the mean BDR for the actual source strength of the wires (0.5 μGyh^{-1}mm^{-1} at 1 m) to give the **implant dose rate:**

   1.3 × 0.5/1.0 = 0.65 Gyh^{-1}

5) Multiply by 85% to **calculate the reference dose rate:**

   0.65 × 0.85 = 0.5525 Gyh^{-1}

6) Divide prescription dose by reference dose rate to **determine treatment time:**

   60/0.5525 = 108.6 hours = 4.5 days

The length of the wires and catheters need to be specified so that there are no underdosed areas at either end of the tumour. To achieve this the catheters or wires must be 20–30% longer than the tumour, this value depends on the wire separation.

The thickness of the volume treated depends on the wire formation and separation:

◆ For a planar formation it is 50–60% of the wire or catheter separation

◆ For a triangular formation it is 120% of the wire or catheter separation

◆ For a square formation it is 150% of the wire or catheter separation.

Paris treatments are based on strict rules and a rigid formation which may be difficult to achieve in the clinic, instead compromises may need to be made, such as finding the average central plane and the average source length for the calculations.

Today, HDR iridium afterloading sources are used instead of iridium wire. Catheters may be placed in the Paris system but calculated with 3D imaging using a TPS and treated with non-uniform dwell patterns to compensate for imperfect catheter arrangements. Particular regions may be boosted in this way, if required.

12.5.2 Manchester gynaecological system

The Manchester system, described in ICRU 38, though originally developed in the 1930s for radium tubes, is still widely used for intracavitary gynaecological treatment for cervical cancer. However, like the Paris system, it is usually now calculated on 3D imaging and then optimized to provide a dose distribution most suitable for the volume being treated. Today, it is most used with HDR afterloader systems.

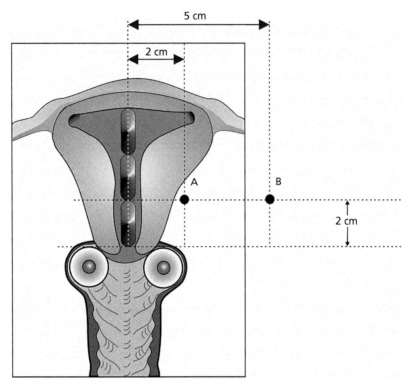

Figure 12.7 Manchester system points definition.
Reproduced with permission from Hoskin and Coyle, Radiotherapy in Practice: Brachytherapy, First Edition, 2005, p. 23, Oxford University Press

The Manchester system describes an intrauterine applicator, rigidly attached to two ovoids that sits in the vaginal fornices (see Figure 12.7). The dose is prescribed to a point with a specific geometric relationship to the applicators, point A is 2 cm superior and 2 cm lateral to the cervical os. The Manchester system dictates that point A must not receive more than one-third of its dose from the vaginal applicator, thus creating a characteristic pear-shaped distribution. An additional reference point is defined, point B: this is representative of the pelvic side wall and is located at the level of point A but 5 cm lateral to the midline. Rectal and bladder dose points are also defined.

The entire setup allows a distribution to be created that is independent of the patient therefore a 'library' plan may be applied which delivers the standardized dose.

In the modern clinic 3D imaging and calculation mean that, whilst a standard Manchester plan may be initially applied, it is often modified or alternatively a plan created from scratch that achieves a distribution with the prescribed dose encompassing the required treatment volume.

12.5.3 **Three-dimensional gynaecological brachytherapy**

The gold standard treatment uses 3D imaging, including MRI for superior soft tissue contrast. The advantages of this are:

- Improved tumour control due to better coverage
- Potential dose escalation
- Improved organ at risk definition and dose minimization
- The ability to accurately sum doses with adjuvant external beam radiotherapy

This technique is set out in the GEC ESTRO guidelines and incorporates the following recommendations:

- Imaging guidelines
- Descriptions of the required target volumes, defined on MRI (e.g. high and intermediate risk clinical target volumes (CTVs))
- Specification of the organs at risk: bladder, rectum, sigmoid, and small bowel
- Dosimetry and dose reporting conventions including:
  - Dose is reported in equivalent 2 Gy doses (EQD2)
  - The minimum dose to 90% and 100% of the CTVs
  - Organs at risk (OAR) doses are reported as the minimum dose to the most irradiated 2 cm^3 and 0.1 cm^3 of the OAR

12.6 **Optimization**

Optimization allows the user to design the dose delivered either by modifying a classic dosimetry system plan or from scratch. It is performed using a treatment planning system, manually and/or via an algorithm.

Patient imaging is imported into the TPS and applicators are reconstructed. Dose objectives (the prescribed tumour doses and organ at risk tolerances) are assigned to either a point, a line, or a volume, depending on the optimization technique. Optimization finds the best spatial and temporal parameters for the sources within those applicators, or the optimization may be performed before the applicators are introduced and, in this case, the optimization will dictate their placement.

12.6.1 **Optimization techniques**

12.6.1.1 Optimize to a reference point

The following points may be defined in the TPS and dose objectives assigned:

- Basal dose points—for Paris-type treatments
- Patient dose points—anatomical points, for example ICRU38 Manchester rectal and bladder points
- Applicator points—at a point of interest or at a specified distance from the applicator

12.6.1.2 Optimize to a reference line

For example, vaginal cylinder HDR brachytherapy:

- Define a reference line at a particular distance from the applicator (e.g. 0.5 cm from cylinder surface)
- Assign an objective that all points on the line receive the prescribed dose

- Equally weighted dwell times would result in a fusiform shaped distribution that is broad at the centre and narrow at the ends
- Through optimization, a cylindrical distribution is achieved by increasing the dwell times at the applicator ends relative to those in the centre (Figures 12.8a and b)
- A library of standard treatment plans, for each cylinder diameter and length, may be designed in this way

12.6.1.3 Optimize to a volume

For example, LDR seed prostate and HDR brachytherapy (commonly prostate and cervix):

- Target and organ at risk structures are delineated on imaging
- Dose-volume objectives are assigned and prioritized, such as:

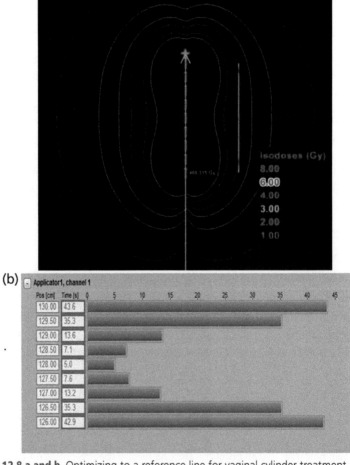

Figure 12.8 a and b Optimizing to a reference line for vaginal cylinder treatment.

- At least 95% of the prescription dose should cover the CTV. Written as V100% > 95%
- No more than 2 cc of rectum should receive the prescribed dose. Written as D2cc < 100% of prescribed dose
- TPS algorithm calculates a source placement plan (either with seeds or HDR stepping source) to best achieve these specifications
- Dose distribution is reviewed and finalized by inspection (Figure 12.9)
- Sources are then delivered in the specified locations

12.6.2 Dose Volume Histograms and dose quality alerts

Dose volume histograms (DVHs, explained in section 9.12.2) are used to analyse the resultant dose distribution. Dose quality alerts may also be set to alert the user if one of the predefined dose-volume objectives has been breached, this is particularly useful when doing real-time planning and treatment, such as a one-stage LDR prostate brachytherapy implant.

12.7 Quality assurance for brachytherapy

Safety is paramount and a well-designed quality assurance (QA) system supports this. QA is integral in every step of the brachytherapy process to ensure the treatment delivered is what was designed, within pre-planned tolerances. Appropriate professional guidance is cited in the Further Reading section. QA differs between delivery modalities, so each will be discussed separately here, broadly each ensures an accuracy of source strength, position, and time.

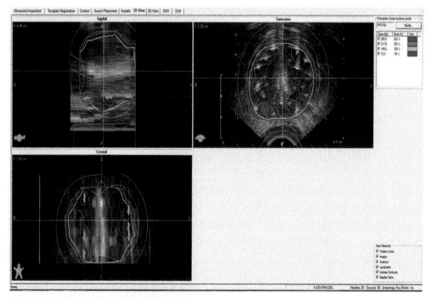

Figure 12.9 Dose distribution from volume optimization—Prostate seed LDR brachytherapy (Varian.com).

12.7.1 Afterloader QA

HDR units, which are the primary means of afterloader brachytherapy in the United Kingdom, are usually subject to a QA programme with a range of checks before each use 'daily QA' and then more in-depth checks at the time of the source being replaced which is usually quarterly for a Ir-192 source. (See Table 12.2).

Additional QA may be required after maintenance and extensive QA must be carried out when new applicators are commissioned including visual and radiographic inspection and characterization of the source path through the applicator.

12.7.2 Manual brachytherapy QA

Manual brachytherapy (for example, prostate seed interstitial LDR brachytherapy) is also subject to a rigorous QA schedule as detailed in Table 12.3.

Table 12.2 HDR afterloader QA tests

Frequency	Test	Method	Tolerance
Daily (Pre-treatment)	Machine function	Emergency equipment, warning signs, interlocks, emergency stop.	
	Applicator and transfer tube integrity	Check applicators and transfer tubes for damage.	
	Position test	Verify source position, using a source viewing jig and CCTV or film.	±1 mm
	Source strength	Ensure that the date time and source strength are correct in the treatment unit and TPS.	±3%
Quarterly (Post source replacement)	Source calibration	RAKR measurement using a well chamber by two independent measurements, traceable to a national standard. Data input into the treatment unit and TPS.	±5%
	Position test	Verify source position, using a source viewing jig and CCTV or film. Source position in an individual applicator may also be characterised.	±2 mm
	Timer test	Check the length of time the source is exposed against an independent stopwatch	±1 s
	Transit time	Ensure that it is consistent and transit dose is low.	
	Applicator and transfer tube integrity	The transfer tubes may be inspected for stretching.	
	Power loss	Check that the source retracts in this event.	
	Leakage radiation	Leakage measured through source housing.	

Table 12.3 Manual brachytherapy QA tests

Frequency	Test	Method	Tolerance
Daily (Pre-treatment)	Source strength	Independent measurement of the source strength is carried out, traceable to a national standard.	±5%
	Connectivity	Between TPS and applicator devices	
	Template grid alignment	Ensure the digital grid aligns with the physical template.	2.0 mm
Varying Frequency	Applicator devices (such as a stepper)	Ensure they are moving and recording their position in an accurate and consistent manner.	0.25 mm and 1.0°
	Verification of activity distribution around a source	An autoradiograph may be used to characterise the source.	
	Leakage Tests	Sources are wiped using water or a solvent and then measured in a scintillation detector to verify whether the source remains sealed.	

12.7.3 TPS QA

QA must also be performed on the treatment planning system, according to the schedule in Table 12.4.

12.7.4 Auxiliary equipment QA

The brachytherapy QA program should also encompass the equipment used to carry out source strength measurements, such as well-type ionization chambers. Checks should be performed annually and cross calibration back to a national standard is recommended every three years. Radiation protection monitors should also be subject to an annual inspection and if appropriate cross-calibration procedure. Other equipment used for handling radioactive sources must also be surveyed regularly and wipe tested (for contamination) if necessary.

12.8 Hazards with sealed sources

An important consideration in any brachytherapy clinic is the safety and storage of the sealed sources. Stringent legislation governs their use including the Ionising Radiation Regulations and the Environmental Permitting Regulations, which are both explored more fully in Chapter 14. It is imperative that the sources are secure, sufficiently shielded, and their location recorded:

◆ Upon receipt, sources should be signed into a central register with details of the source and its storage location.

◆ The sources' secure storage needs to be regularly audited to ensure accuracy of inventory.

Table 12.4 Treatment planning system QA tests

Frequency	Test	Method	Tolerance
Daily (Pre-treatment)	Plan transfer	Checks should be made that the plan has transferred to the TPS correctly and source strength and dwell times are as expected.	
	Plan check	Individual treatment plans are independently checked, including a source data check and a dose calculation is made either by hand or independent software.	±5%
	Data file integrity	Using check-sum methodology.	
Varying frequently	Image acquisition	Any imaging used for source placement, treatment planning or verification must also be subject to its own QA schedule.	
	Image registration	Registration between images is assessed.	
	Geometric reconstruction	This ensures that the applicators are reconstructed accurately in all imaging modalities.	
	End to end testing	This tests the entire planning process from start to finish and may form part of an audit.	
	Complex dosimetry tests	Complex plans may be created and independent dose calculations made	
	On screen calculation and display	Isodoses and DVHs may be analysed.	

- Wipe testing should be performed on all sources annually.
- A robust system needs to be implemented that records source movement, ideally with a log in both locations.
- Additional consideration is needed if the source is to be transported off site.
- Safe disposal of sources entails financial implications and should be considered before acquisition.
- Staff should be trained in safe retrieval of dislodged sources. Appropriate equipment, including long-handled forceps, a shielded container and radiation monitor, should be always made available.

Appendix 12-A: Determination of reference air kerma rate

Measuring RAKR

RAKR may be measured in the clinic by following the advice in the relevant approved code of practice. The source is introduced to a well-type ionization chamber, either manually or using the afterloader. The location of maximal current reading, known as the 'sweet spot' is determined, then measurements are taken at this location. RAKR is usually measured in the department before a source is used and as part of the quality assurance (QA) schedule.

$$\text{RAKR } (\mu Gy \ m^2 \ h^{-1}) = \text{Mean current (A)} \times N_{k,R} \times f_{ion} \times f_{elec} \times f_{tp}$$

$N_{k,R}$ is the air kerma chamber calibration factor provided by calibration at a national standards laboratory.

f_{ion} is the ion recombination factor

f_{elec} is the electrometer correction factor

f_{tp} is the temperature and pressure correction factor

RAKR to dose—point source

Once the RAKR has been determined it is then necessary to look at how this translates to dose delivered. These calculations may be done by hand, or by the TPS. One of the simplest ways to determine the dose from a given RAKR is to assume the source is a point (i.e. has no physical dimensions). Professional guidance gives the following equation:

$$Dose \ at \ a \ distance, r = RAKR \times \frac{(\frac{\mu}{\rho})water}{(\frac{\mu}{\rho})air} \times \left(\frac{r_{ref}}{r}\right)^2 \times F \times t$$

$\frac{(\frac{\mu}{\rho})water}{(\frac{\mu}{\rho})air}$ is the ratio of mass energy absorption co-efficients which converts AKR to dose in water (varies for different sources).

$\left(\frac{r_{ref}}{r}\right)^2$ corrects for the distance to the measurement point from the reference distance.

F corrects for the attenuation and scatter in tissue, from published experimental data in water

t is the treatment time (how long the source is in place).

RAKR to dose—cylindrical source

RAKR was further refined to introduce the concept of air kerma strength, S_K, defined as the product of the air kerma at distance d measured along the transverse bisector of the source and the square of distance d. This is measured in U, which is equivalent to 1 μGym^2h^{-1}.

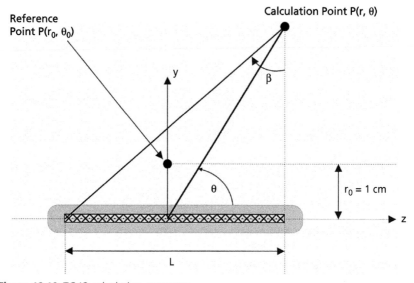

Figure 12.10 TG43 calculation geometry.
Reproduced with permission from Hoskin and Coyle, Radiotherapy in Practice: Brachytherapy, First Edition, 2005, p. 39, Oxford University Press

This equation describes the dose from a cylindrical source (Figure 12.10), which is more representative of the real-life situation and is the method in use in many brachytherapy TPSs today.

$$Dose\,rate\,at\,a\,point, P = S_k \times \Delta \times \left(\frac{G(r,\theta)}{G(r_0,\theta_0)} \right) \times g(r) \times F(r,\theta)$$

where

Δ is the Dose Rate Constant in water, it is the dose rate to water at 1 cm on the transverse axis of a source of 1 U and includes the effects of source geometry, spatial distribution of radioactivity, encapsulation, self-filtration by the source, and scattering.

$\left(\frac{G(r,\theta)}{G(r_0,\theta_0)} \right)$ is the geometry function, this accounts for the dose variation due only to the spatial distribution of radioactivity within the source.

$g(r)$ is the radial dose function, this accounts for the dose rate fall-off along the transverse axis due to absorption and scattering in the medium. It may be likened to depth dose in external beam radiotherapy.

$F(r,\theta)$ is the anisotropy function, this accounts for the anisotropy of the dose distribution around the source, including the effects of self-filtration, oblique filtration of primary photons through the encapsulating material, internal scattering within the source, and attenuation and scattering in the surrounding water medium.

Model-based dose calculation algorithms

So far, the RAKR to dose calculations have assumed that the dose is being delivered to water, this is not a surprising assumption given the electron density of human tissue is largely equivalent to water and the assumption is correct within a certain accuracy, especially for pelvic applications.

Modern treatment planning systems use electron density information from a CT scan to model the dose distribution more accurately. Heterogeneities in tissue can alter the brachytherapy dose distribution quite significantly and whilst accounting for inhomogeneities for external beam planning has been common for many years, for brachytherapy it is a recent introduction but is set to pave the way for more accurate brachytherapy dose calculations in the future.

Chapter 13

Molecular radiotherapy

Jonathan Gear, Brenda Pratt, and Glenn Flux

13.1 Introduction

Unsealed sources of radioactivity have been used for the treatment of benign and malignant conditions for over 80 years. They can be given orally in liquid or capsule form, by intravenous or intra-arterial infusion, or by direct injection into tumours or body cavities. The term 'molecular radiotherapy' (MRT) is increasingly used to indicate that this is a form of systemic radiotherapy for which treatment outcome is dependent on the absorbed doses delivered to tumours or target volumes and to organs at risk (OAR). A large range of radiotherapeutics are used for a variety of indications.

The clinical aspects of MRT have been extensively covered in a previous book in this series (*Radiotherapy in Practice: Radioisotope Therapy*), therefore this chapter will focus on the main physics aspects only.

13.2 Treatment planning

In common with external beam radiotherapy (EBRT), treatment planning can be used to optimize effectiveness and to ensure that the absorbed doses delivered to healthy organs are within limits that will avoid unacceptable toxicity. Treatment planning parameters for MRT may be considered separately in terms of the radiotherapeutic that is used, that is the radionuclide and the pharmaceutical, and how it is administered regarding the level of activity and the frequency of administration.

13.2.1 Choice of radiotherapeutic

The optimal choice of radiotherapeutic for MRT is dependent on physical properties including the type of radiation emissions, their range in tissue, the linear energy transfer, the chemical properties that are required for localization, and the physical half-life that determines retention in the organ under investigation as well as the dose rate.

13.2.2 Types of emission

Most radionuclide treatments use beta particle emitters, for example iodine as ^{131}I for thyroid disorders and lutetium as ^{177}Lu in peptide receptor therapy. More recently, the use of alpha emitting radionuclides has increased, particularly with the approval of radium as ^{223}Ra for the treatment of castrate-resistant prostate cancer metastatic to bone. Treatment planning for MRT is aided by the using radionuclides that emit gamma rays of suitable energy for detection and imaging to assess the distribution and/or uptake of the radiopharmaceutical. However, the presence of gamma radiation increases the absorbed dose delivered to normal tissues and requires increased precautions related to radiation protection. Pure beta emitters, including phosphorus as ^{32}P and yttrium as ^{90}Y, offer the potential to image or externally measure the bremsstrahlung radiation produced.

13.2.3 **Range in tissue**

Ideally the range of the particles will be matched to the size of the lesions being treated. The range of a particle depends on its energy. Therefore, if the particle energy is high and the lesion size small some of the particle energy may be deposited outside the lesion causing a reduction in absorbed dose to the lesion and unnecessary dose to normal tissue. Conversely, in a larger tumour exhibiting a pronounced degree of heterogeneous uptake, a longer-range beta emitter will irradiate a larger proportion of viable cells due to crossfire. Auger electrons have a very short range (generally < 1 μm) and are therefore only of use when attached or very close to the cell nucleus. Alpha particles have a range equivalent to several cell diameters (typically 50–90 μm). Beta emissions from ^{131}I or ^{177}Lu have a range of 1–3 mm while the pure beta emitters ^{90}Y and ^{32}P have a maximum range in tissue of approximately 1 cm. The typical range of such particles is illustrated in Figure 13.1.

13.2.4 **Linear energy transfer and specific ionization**

A charged particle travelling through a medium loses energy and produces ionization. The linear energy transfer (LET) of particles has been discussed in sections 2.6.4 and 3.3.2. Particles with high values of LET are important for radionuclide therapy as they cause more biological damage to a cell than those with low values. Values for alpha particles are typically 100 times greater than for electrons of the same energy.

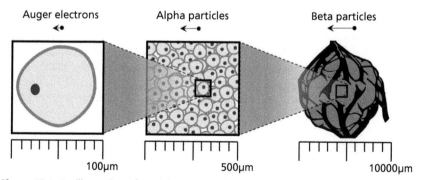

Figure 13.1 An illustration of particle range with respect to typical tissue and cell dimensions.

13.2.5 **Chemical properties**

The chemical properties of a radiopharmaceutical determine its behaviour in the body. Radiopharmaceuticals are designed for maximum uptake in the tumours or normal organs of interest and minimum uptake elsewhere in the body, so they must remain chemically stable for as long as possible. The shelf life of a radiopharmaceutical, quoted as time after an activity reference date, is stated by the manufacturer. Example shelf lives for therapy radiopharmaceuticals are two to six weeks for ^{131}I NaI capsules and two days for ^{131}I mIBG (metaiodobenzylguanidine). There may be other stipulations for product preparation. For example, m^{131}IBG delivered frozen must be used within two hours of defrosting and dilution. Radiopharmaceuticals prepared in-house have no specific shelf life (e.g. many antibody and peptide preparations) and must undergo stringent quality control testing before use. If the shelf life of a product is exceeded, then the radiopharmaceutical will become chemically unstable. This will result in non-specific uptake of radioactivity in the body and unwanted radiation dose in these areas. It is important to note that even where shelf life is relatively long, the radio-nuclide will decay physically during this time and the activity remaining may be too low for effective clinical use. Drug interactions must also be considered as chemical interactions may affect the behaviour of the radiopharmaceutical. Therefore, it may be necessary to alter the patient's medication prior to administration.

13.2.6 **Activity**

The activity, A, of a radionuclide is the rate that nuclear decays or transition occur, and can be written as

$$A = \frac{dN}{dt} = -\lambda N.$$

(13.1)

Where N is the number of nuclei at that instant, t is time, and λ is the decay constant which has units of s^{-1} and represents the proportion of N that decay in one second. As N is continually decreasing over time, the activity, A_t after some time, t, can be expressed as

$$A_t = A_{t=0}e^{-\lambda t}$$

(13.2)

The unit of activity is the becquerel (Bq), where 1 Bq is equivalent to one decay per second. The curie (Ci) is still sometimes used, where; 1 Ci = 37,000,000 Bq or 37 MBq. In diagnostic nuclear medicine the activity is of the order of 100 MBq (100×10^6). For therapy most administered activities are in the order of a few GBq (1×10^9). Therapies using alpha emitters generally use significantly lower activities, in the order of 80 kBq per kilogram body weight.

13.2.7 **Half-life**

The physical half-life, T_p of a radionuclide is the time taken for the activity to decay to half of its original value and can be expressed in terms of lambda

$$T_p = \frac{\ln(2)}{\lambda} \tag{13.3}$$

The biological half-life of a pharmaceutical in a region of the body is the time taken for that drug to reduce to half of its original concentration, due to biological excretion. The effective half-life of a radiopharmaceutical, within a tumour, organ, or the (T_e) is dependent on both the physical (T_p) and biological (T_b) half-lives as shown in Equation 13.4. This can be measured directly using either quantitative imaging or external radiation counting.

$$\frac{1}{T_e} = \frac{1}{T_p} + \frac{1}{T_b} \tag{13.4}$$

13.2.8 Dose rate

In contrast to external beam radiotherapy, radionuclide therapy delivers continuous irradiation at low and ever decreasing dose rates. An absorbed dose has a reduced biological effect if delivered at low dose rate as the irradiated cells have more time to repair damage between ionizations. Tissues that respond quickly to irradiation, such as cancer cells and bone marrow, are less affected by this reduction in dose rate than later responding tissues, such as the kidney. The overall effect is the sparing of late responding healthy tissues in the later stages of therapy, thereby maximizing the differential sparing between tumour and normal tissues. The dose rate in a particular tumour or organ during therapy varies according to the effective half-life of the radio-activity in that volume.

13.3 Dosimetry techniques

The IR(ME)R 2017 regulations state that all radiation exposures should be individually planned and that the radiation delivery should be verified after administration. Radiation doses delivered to normal tissues should be kept as low as reasonably practicable (ALARP). Traditionally, most radionuclide therapy procedures are prescribed to standard levels of activity without regard to or calculation of the delivered absorbed dose. However, there is now increasing evidence of correlations between the delivered absorbed dose distribution and outcome in terms of response and toxicity. There is therefore an opportunity to perform personalized dosimetry for all patients to both record and optimize the treatment.

Individualized dosimetry-based treatment planning may be performed either from pre-therapy tracer studies or from an ongoing 'adaptive' process for multicycle treatments. For pre-therapy tracer studies a low activity of the therapy radiopharmaceutical is administered to the patient and dosimetry measurements carried out. The doses delivered to tumours and organs of interest are then calculated and the amount of activity to be administered for therapy is determined, under the assumption that the absorbed dose will scale linearly with the activity given. The tracer and therapy administrations should occur close in time (although for ^{131}I NaI treatment of thyroid disease there is a possibility of reduced therapy uptake due to 'stunning' if they are too close together). The pre-therapy study may alternatively use a companion diagnostic radioisotope more suited to quantitative imaging. Examples include ^{123}I mIBG or ^{124}I mIBG SPECT (single photon emission computed tomography) studies before therapy with ^{131}I mIBG, and ^{111}In DOTATATE SPECT before ^{90}Y or ^{177}Lu DOTATATE therapy for the treatment of neuroendocrine disease.

An adaptive approach to treatment planning is becoming more prevalent and may be considered when multiple administrations are given as a course of treatment. In this case, the activity for the first therapy might be decided empirically or from a weight-based formula. Absorbed doses are then calculated after each administration and used to modify the next treatment.

The most widely used framework to calculate absorbed doses was developed by the Medical Internal Radiation Dose (MIRD) committee of the Society for Nuclear Medicine. Although originally developed for diagnostic nuclear medicine, the MIRD schema are work well for therapy.

13.3.1 MIRD schema

In the MIRD system, the body is considered to be composed of *source organs* that exhibit uptake of radioactivity and *target organs* for which the absorbed dose is to be calculated. Frequently in therapeutic procedures the aim is to calculate the *self-dose* because the source and target organs are the same. The total number of radioactive disintegrations that occur in the source organ, $\tilde{A}_S$, are given by the area under the time-activity curve measured following administration, and termed time-integrated activity. This is given by

$$\tilde{A}_S = \int_0^\infty A_{S,t}dt, \tag{13.5}$$

where $A_{S,t}$ is the activity remaining in a source organ, S, at time t. While the absorbed dose can be calculated for any given period, the limits are usually taken to be from the time of administration to infinity so that the total absorbed dose is calculated.

The mean energy emitted per nuclear disintegration depends on the energy and frequency of the emissions. For an emission i of radiation of type alpha, beta, or gamma, this is termed the equilibrium absorbed dose constant, Δ_i. The fraction of the energy of i emitted from the source and absorbed by the target is called the absorbed fraction, ϕ_i. This depends not only on the type and energy of the emission, but also on ϕ_i being 1 when the source and target organs are the same and 0 when source and target organs are physically separated.

Once the parameters described above have been determined the following equation is used to calculate the absorbed dose, $D_{t\leftarrow s}$ (in Gy), to the target organ from the activity in the source organ:

$$D_{t\leftarrow s} = \frac{\tilde{A}_S}{m_t}\sum_i \Delta_i\phi_i \tag{13.6}$$

where $\tilde{A}_S$ (in MBq.h), Δ_i (in g Gy MBq^{-1} h^{-1}) and ϕ_i are as defined above and m_t is the mass of the target organ in g.

The mean dose per unit time-integrated activity, $\dfrac{1}{m_t}\sum_i \Delta_i \phi_i$ is known as the S value and Equation 13.6 simplifies to:

$$D_{t\leftarrow s} = \tilde{A}_s S_{t\leftarrow s} \tag{13.7}$$

In general, there will be multiple source organs in the body and the total dose to each target organ is simply the sum of the contributions to each target from the individual source organs.

13.3.2 MIRD calculations in practice

13.3.2.1 Determination of time-integrated activity, $\tilde{A}_s$

To calculate the time integrated activity in a source organ, it is necessary to determine the activity in the organ at multiple time points following administration of the radionuclide. In practice, there are several ways to measure the activity, as discussed in sections 13.4 and 13.5, and to generate an activity time curve. To describe the curve accurately it is vital to ensure that the number and frequency of the activity measurements are adequate. The time-integrated activity is equal to the area under the time-activity curve which in the case of a single organ or lesion, can often be expressed as a single exponential:

$$A_S(t) = A_{S,t=0}e^{-\lambda t} \tag{13.8}$$

where the uptake in the organ is assumed to be instantaneous at time $A_{S,t=0}$.

Using Equations 13.5 and 13.8, the time-integrated activity may be expressed as

$$\tilde{A}_s = \frac{A_{S,t=0} \cdot T_e}{\ln(2)} \tag{13.9}$$

In some cases the time-activity curve may be more complex and is described by the combination of more than one exponential, either as uptake or excretion phases.

13.3.3 Determination of S values (and mass of target organ, m_t)

S values have been tabulated for a variety of radionuclides and for different models of source-target combinations and calculated using standard human phantoms. These models are designed to represent standard human geometries. Examples include a standard 70 kg man, children of various ages, and women at different stages of gestation. If the anatomy of the patient does not match those of the model, corrections may be applied by scaling by the ratio of phantom and patient organ mass. Patient organ volumes may be measured with high resolution imaging such as ultrasound, computed tomography (CT), or magnetic resonance imaging (MRI). Alternatively, SPECT or positron emission tomography (PET) may be used to estimate a functional volume, but these will have relatively poor spatial resolution. As tumours do not have standardized geometry, S values for spherical volumes are conventionally used.

13.3.4 Limitations of the MIRD scheme

The MIRD schema has its limitations. The assumption is made that the radioactivity is uniformly distributed in the source organ which is unlikely to be the case in practice. A further assumption is that the organ sizes and shapes in the patient are the same as those in the standard human phantoms used in the scheme. In addition, only a mean absorbed dose in the target organ is calculated, despite the possibility that the maximum and minimum doses may differ significantly from this. Nevertheless, the MIRD system itself is elegant, as accurate as the input data allow, and highly practical.

13.3.5 Dose-limiting organs

As in EBRT, the absorbed doses delivered to the normal organs limit the maximum absorbed dose that can be delivered to target volumes. In systemic radionuclide therapy the dose-limiting organ is usually the bone marrow. Doses to normal organs can be reduced, for example by giving amino acids and diuretics to reduce kidney dose in ^{177}Lu DOTATATE therapy, or by hydration to reduce bladder dose. A bone marrow harvest may be taken before therapy for regrafting after therapy if necessary. Extensive dosimetry and toxicity studies are essential to determine the dose-limiting organs for new therapy agents.

13.4 *In-vivo* activity estimation

Activity quantification can be performed using a variety of different measurement and imaging systems. The simplest approach is to use an external probe, such as Geiger counter or scintillation monitor, to measure the activity in the whole-body. Quantitative SPECT/PET/CT systems can use hybrid imaging and tomography to determine uptake and retention in individual organs and tissues. The choice of system to use will depend on the radionuclide and emissions, and on factors such as equipment availability and acceptable measurement time. Regardless of the system used, there will be aspects of the measurement procedure that introduce uncertainty in the final activity estimation. It is therefore necessary to avoid, reduce or correct for these effects during the quantification process. The most important issues to be considered in measurement and imaging for dosimetry are outlined below.

13.4.1 Acquisition time

The acquisition or imaging period must be long enough to enable adequate emissions to be detected, but not so long as to be uncomfortable for the patient. The percentage error in the recorded count reduces with increasing events according to Poisson statistics.

13.4.2 Dead time

All systems have an inherent dead-time which is the length of time a system takes to process an event after detection, during which no further events can be processed. A substantial proportion of true events may be lost if the count rate incident on a detector is high. This is particularly an issue for imaging therapeutic levels of I-131. Corrections are needed to account for this loss to enable accurate activity quantification.

13.4.3 System sensitivity

To calculate time-integrated activity, the events acquired in the detector must be converted into corresponding levels of activity using a sensitivity factor. The calibration method is generally used in whole body measurements with Geiger counters. Emission events from the patient are counted immediately after the radiopharmaceutical administration and before their first void. As no activity has been excreted, the calibration factor is simply the recorded count rate divided by the administered activity. Subsequent count rates from the patient are multiplied by this factor to convert them to activity levels. In the case of SPECT, it is common to scan a phantom representative of the patient that contains one or more radio-active sources of known activity and volume representing the tumours (or normal organs) of interest. The scan is performed with identical scan parameters to the patient scan. After appropriate corrections have been made to the images (as outlined above), the counts in the patient and phantom images are determined. The counts within a given region of the patient scan are converted to activity by multiplication of the calibration factor which is given by the phantom counts divided by the phantom activity.

13.4.4 SPECT vs planar imaging

Both 2-dimensional (planar) and 3-dimensional (SPECT) imaging have been used for activity quantification. A SPECT scan will have poorer resolution than the equivalent planar scans, but offers the major advantage of providing 3D data with improved contrast. 3D data are considered essential for accurate dosimetry to determine the precise pattern of activity uptake and to assess changes in distribution over time. SPECT/CT and PET/CT scans are useful in this respect. Planar imaging may be more applicable where the count rates are too low for SPECT, and if there is little concern of activity contained in under- or over-lying tissue.

13.4.5 Attenuation and scatter

Radiation passing through a medium will be attenuated and scattered by the medium. Corrections for attenuation and scatter minimize degradation of image quality and errors in quantification. Methods range in complexity from the use of scatter windows during gamma camera imaging to the generation of correction maps from registered CT image and Monte Carlo simulations performed during image reconstruction.

13.4.6 Registration

To determine how the activity distribution in the body changes over time it is often necessary to register sets of scans to each other. This can include registration of sequential SPECT images or registration of SPECT with CT (section 8.6).

13.5 **Examples for interest**

13.5.1 ^{131}I NaI for treatment of hyperthyroidism

The following example can be used to prescribe the ^{131}I activity required to restore a patient with Graves' disease to euthyroid status. According to European Association of Nuclear Medicine guidelines this requires approximately 150 Gy. A tracer administration of 0.2 MBq of ^{131}I in capsule form was planned for administration to predict the biological uptake and retention in the thyroid.

A sodium iodine detector coupled to a multichannel analyser and energy discriminator was used for the task. The detector was shielded and suitably collimated to detect emissions from only the thyroid bed at 10 cm. To calibrate the detection system the ^{131}I capsule was first positioned within a Perspex neck phantom 10 cm from the detector and emission data collected for a period of 10 minutes. After administration, 5-minute acquisitions were acquired of the patient's thyroid at 2, 4, 24, 48, 120, and 192 hours post administration.

The detector recorded 60,000 counts during the calibration measurement giving a sensitivity factor of 500 cps/MBq. The measured count rate and calculated activity in the thyroid are summarized in Table 13.1. A fit of percentage activity in the thyroid as a function of time, accounting for uptake and a single decay phase, is shown in Figure 13.2. For ease of calculation, a single exponential function was assumed, ignoring the first two data points. This approximation results in an overestimation of absorbed dose of approximately 1%.

From Figure 13.2 the effective half-life, $T_e = 156$ h and $A_{S,t=0} = 0.142$ MBq. Therefore, using Equation 13.9, the time-integrated activity is

$$\tilde{A}_s = \frac{A_{S,t=0} \cdot T_e}{\ln(2)} = 31.96 \text{ MBq.h} \qquad (13.10)$$

In MIRD pamphlet 11, the S-value for a model thyroid, of mass, $m_{model} = 19.63$ g is given as 5.95×10^{-3} Gy/MBq.h. The patient thyroid mass, $m_{patient}$, had previously been determined using ultrasound to be 30 g. A scaling to the S-value is therefore applied;

$$S_{patient} = \frac{m_{model}}{m_{patient}} S_{phantom} = 3.89 \times 10^{-3} \text{ Gy MBq}^{-1}\text{h}^{-1} \qquad (13.11)$$

Table 13.1 Table of thyroid uptake values measured using the thyroid counter

Time post admin (hrs)	Count rate	Activity (MBq)
2	25.9	0.05
4	29.91	0.06
24	62.48	0.13
48	55.11	0.11
120	40.05	0.08
192	30.13	0.06

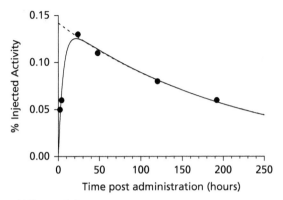

Figure 13.2 Thyroid time activity curve.

Using Equation 13.7 giving the absorbed dose from the 0.2 MBq tracer administration is

$$\bar{D} = \tilde{A}_s S_{patient} = 0.124\ Gy \tag{13.12}$$

Therefore, to deliver a prescribed absorbed dose of 150 Gy, an administered activity of 241 MBq of ^{131}I NaI is required.

13.5.2 Lu-177 DOTATATE dosimetry during therapy

In this example, the absorbed dose from a 7.4 GBq administration of Lu-177 DOTATATE is calculated and used to predict the cumulative absorbed dose for a full four-cycle treatment. SPECT/CT images were acquired at 24, 48, and 72 hours post administration. A large neuroendocrine tumour measuring approximately 11 cm in diameter involving liver segments IVb and V is the focus of the dosimetry calculation. The images were reconstructed and corrected for scatter and attenuation effects using the CT data. The lesion was delineated using the anatomical CT data and found to measure 274 ml. The delineated volume was copied to the registered SPECT series and the counts within the volume converted to activity using a pre acquired sensitivity factor of 10.5 cps/MBq. A previous phantom study demonstrated that count losses due to partial volume effects are approximately 20% for this sized volume.

The activity in the lesion was calculated using

$$A_t = \frac{C_t}{Q.R} \tag{13.13}$$

Where C_t is the count rate within the lesion volume at time t, Q is the sensitivity factor and R is the recovery factor equal to 0.8. A fused SPECT/CT image with delineated volume is given in Figure 13.3a, maximum intensity projections at each of the time points are given in Figure 13.3b, c, and d. The derived time activity curve is given in Figure 13.4a.

(a)   (b)   (c)   (d)

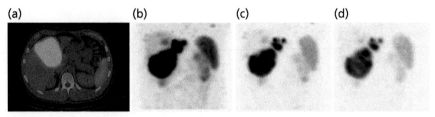

Figure 13.3 SPECT/CT image demonstrating uptake in large liver lesion (a), with maximum intensity projections images acquired are 24 (b), 24 (c), and 72 hours (d) post administration.

Similarly with the previous example, an exponential function with and without an uptake phase can be fitted to the data. As no data were acquired before 24 hours it is not possible to ascertain which of the two curves more accurately represents the biokinetics of the radiopharmaceutical. For the case of instantaneous lesion uptake the effective half-life, $T_e = 41.4$ h and $A_{S,t=0} = 1537$ MBq. Therefore, using Equation 13.9, the time-integrated activity is

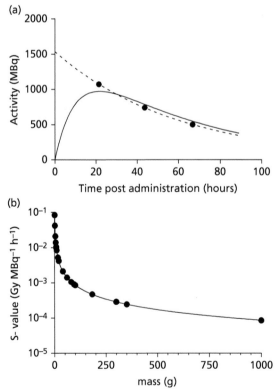

Figure 13.4 Lesion time activity curve showing two potential fits to the data (a). A plot of S-values for different sized spheres of unit density (b).

$$\tilde{A}_s = \frac{A_s(0).T_e}{\ln(2)} = 91761 \text{ MBq.h}$$ (13.14)

The time-integrated activity using the function with the uptake phase would be 83503 *MBq.h*

S-value data for the lesion were extrapolated from the unit density sphere models within the OLINDA/EXM software. These have been plotted in Figure 13.4b. Assuming unit tissue density within the lesion, an S-value of 3.16×10^{-4} Gy/MBq.h is used.

Using Equation 13.7, the absorbed dose from the first Lu-177 DOTATATE cycle is therefore between 26 Gy and 29 Gy, depending on how the time-activity curve is fitted. Assuming a similar uptake and retention pattern for the subsequent cycles, the cumulative lesion absorbed dose is expected to be between 106 Gy and 116 Gy. The uncertainty in this dose measurement could be decreased if earlier imaging time points were acquired so that the rate of tracer uptake was ascertained more accurately.

Chapter 14

Radiation protection in radiotherapy

Jim Thurston

14.1 Introduction

The aim of radiation protection is to minimize the risk of harm whilst retaining the benefit of the use of ionizing radiation. Radiation protection practices must predict both the benefit and the harm from a given radiation dose, and to be able to quantify both for direct comparison, at a reasonable cost. We also need to account for natural sources of ionizing radiation contributing to human exposure, and deliberate uses must therefore be set into context to that overall exposure.

14.2 Sources of ionizing radiation exposure—natural and artificial

Life on Earth has evolved whilst being exposed to a range of sources of ionizing radiation, giving a small but measurable radiation dose; this is called natural background radiation. There are then the other sources of exposure which are 'artificial' or human-made.

The natural background radiation, which is mostly unavoidable, arises from natural radioactivity in the ground, cosmic rays from space, atmospheric radon, other radioactive gases as decay products of radioactivity in the environment, and from natural radioactivity in foodstuffs.

Artificial sources include the medical uses of ionizing radiation, occupational exposure, discharges of radionuclides to the environment from nuclear power generation, and fallout from the nuclear weapons tests carried out in the mid-late twentieth century.

N.B. Doses quoted are effective doses in milliSievert (mSv)—see Section 14.5.1.

For the average person in the United Kingdom (Table 14.1), natural background radiation constitutes the most significant contribution to their exposure, however medical exposure, even when averaged over the whole population (most of whom do not receive an X-ray or other medical exposure), still provides the most significant artificial contribution to the total radiation dose. In most cases it isn't practicable to attempt to reduce the population exposure to natural sources, but it is possible and desirable to reduce the doses received to as low as reasonably practicable from those practices involving ionizing radiation—especially medical uses.

Table 14.1 Annual radiation doses to the UK population

	Average dose per person (mSv)	**Percentage contribution (%)**
Natural		
Cosmic	0.33	11.9
Gamma rays	0.35	13.1
Internal radionuclides	0.27	10.1
Radon	1.3	48.7
SUBTOTAL Natural	2.25	83.7
Artificial		
Medical	0.44	16.0
Occupational	0.0004	0.02
Fallout	0.005	0.18
Disposals	0.0008	0.03
SUBTOTAL Artificial	0.446	16.3
TOTAL (Rounded)	2.7	100

That is the main goal of radiation protection. First though we should consider what is known about the effects of exposure to ionizing radiation, and where that knowledge comes from.

14.3 Effects of ionizing radiation and sources of data

It is useful to outline the basic categorization of the biological effects of radiation (radiobiology), based on the mechanisms for the damage caused, and on whether the damage caused is either *deterministic* or *stochastic*.

The damage mechanisms can be described as follows:

14.3.1 Direct action

Direct action occurs when the ionizing radiation interacts directly with the DNA in the cell—in other words that an ionization occurs causing a co-valent electron to be ejected from an atom within the DNA molecular chain. This causes a break in the DNA, whether on the double strands or the base pairs. The ionization event has *directly* led to a biological effect in this case.

14.3.2 Indirect action

Indirect action occurs when the ionizing event occurs within the cytoplasm or other molecules within the cell rather than with the DNA directly. The ionization may cause, for example, the breaking of a water molecule (H_2O) into free radical forms of hydrogen and oxygen. These are chemically very reactive; they may combine back to H_2O in which case it is likely that no harm has been done. However, they may instead recombine as other molecules which are hazardous to the cell, such as OH, or H_2O_2. The presence of these in the cell may then lead to biological damage. So the initial action of ionization has caused a chemical reaction that then *indirectly* leads to a biological effect.

We can classify the resulting deleterious biological effects themselves based on the severity or the probability of the effect occurring, as follows.

14.3.3 Deterministic effects

These occur at higher radiation doses as a consequence of cell death, which for the most part are relatively immediate (also termed 'early' or 'acute'). They *definitely* occur in all persons exposed to such radiation doses. The early effects lead to rapid injury, necrosis of a tissue and thus through consequent localized damage potentially to the loss of function of organs and the death of the whole organism. Some of these effects and others can occur a long time after the initial exposure. Deterministic effects only occur at high doses with a severity increasing with the dose received. There is also a threshold dose below which effects are not seen—the reason being that RNA and other proteins and enzymes carry out repair on the damaged DNA within each cell, and cells are in any case being replaced at different rates based on cell/tissue type. Thus if the radiation dose received is below a certain level, cell repair and replacement occur at a faster rate than cell death and consequently no effect is observed. Conversely, if cell death occurs at a faster rate than repair or replacement due to higher doses received, then the effects observed worsen as the dose is increased. Although still subject to individual variability to the doses received, the tissue responses above the threshold are predictable and can be studied experimentally or clinically, and International Commission on Radiation Protection (ICRP) prefer nowadays to refer to deterministic effects as '*tissue reactions*' (see Figure 14.1a).

The dose at which effects are first observed is known as the threshold dose, which will be determined by the type of tissue, and in terms of absorbed dose (see Chapter 5) ranges from a few tenths of a Gray up to several Gray (see Table 14.2 for examples). Some adverse effects can be temporary rather than permanent.

14.3.4 Stochastic effects

Stochastic effects are as a result of processes that are governed by chance. Ionizing radiation can interact with the DNA of the cell nucleus; where damage cannot be repaired the effect will be manifested as a mutation which can lead to cancer or hereditary disease after several cell divisions and the passage of time. It should be noted that damage to DNA may mean that the cell suspends its cycle, does not go to mitosis, and so there is no consequent effect. Also note that the time for a cancer to develop could be many years after the initial exposure. For leukaemias the minimum time (called the latency period) between the exposure and diagnosis can be from 2–10 years, and for solid tumours can be from 5 to over 30 years. This is important when considering such effects occurring in different aged groups in the exposed population (see Section 14.6). The features of deterministic and stochastic effects are summarized in Box 14.1.

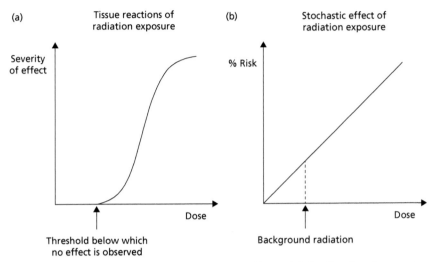

Figure 14.1 Response curves for (a) tissue reactions (deterministic effects) and (b) stochastic effects.
Reproduced from Moreels M. et al. (2020) 'Stress and Radiation Responsiveness'. In: Choukèr A. (eds) Stress Challenges and Immunity in Space. Springer, Cham. under a Creative Commons Attribution 4.0 International License (http://creativecommons.org/licenses/by/4.0/)

Table 14.2 Threshold doses (absorbed dose) for deterministic effects

Tissue and effect:	Received in a single brief exposure (Gy)	Received in highly fractionated or protracted exposures (Gy)	Received yearly in highly fractionated or protracted exposures for many years (Gy y⁻¹)
Threshold Dose:			
Testes:			
- Temporary sterility	0.15	NA	0.4
- Permanent sterility	3.5–6.0	NA	2.0
Ovaries:			
- Sterility	2.5–6.0	6.0	> 0.2
Lens:			> 0.1
- Detectable opacities	0.5–2.0	5	> 0.15
- Visual impairment (Cataract)	5.0	>8	
Bone marrow:			
- Depression of haematopoiesis	0.5	NA	> 0.4

Box 14.1 Summary of effects

Harmful tissue reactions—i.e. deterministic effects:

- ◆ Only occur when the threshold dose is exceeded
- ◆ Become more severe with increasing dose
- ◆ Occur relatively soon after exposure

Stochastic effects:

- ◆ Might occur at any radiation dose, however small (no threshold)
- ◆ Only the likelihood, not severity, increases as the dose increases
- ◆ May occur many years after the exposure

The important feature of stochastic effects is that they can occur as a consequence of doses which are very much lower than those that can cause deterministic damage. Indeed, it is believed that there is no threshold dose below which they cannot occur, although this is difficult to prove and is not accepted universally. Furthermore, only the probability (or risk), not the outcome, can be predicted from the dose. For the individual concerned, the probability of the event is small, but its effect may be life-changing, or possibly fatal. The general stochastic response to radiation dose is represented in Figure 14.1b.

14.3.4.1 The evidence for deterministic and stochastic effects

Over the last century, there have been many studies that establish a causal relationship between exposure to ionizing radiation and the induction of cancer.

These include:

- ◆ occupational exposure,
- ◆ medical diagnosis,
- ◆ medical therapy, and
- ◆ use and testing of atomic bombs.

14.3.5 Occupational exposure

The first evidence of the harmful effects of radiation came from observations on workers exposed to ionizing radiation. They included of course the pioneers in the science of radiation physics and its application to medicine. A classic example of occupational exposure was presented in Chapter 3, discussing the women employed by the US Radium Corporation. Although this provided evidence of the carcinogenic effects of radiation, inadequate dosimetry prevented the derivation of risk estimates.

Studies of uranium miners have demonstrated the effects of breathing radon in the higher concentrations found in mines. These have provided some of the best data on the risk estimates from high linear energy transfer (LET) radiation such as alpha particles.

Examination of mortality and disease statistics for workers monitored for radiation exposure has also potentially been the best data source for risks from low levels of ionizing radiation. However, there are a number of practical difficulties: the inadequate sample size, incomplete time for full incidence to be observed, potential confounding effects, and the 'healthy worker' effect. From the 1980s the UK National Registry of Radiation Workers (NRRW) enrolled the records of about 100,000 workers and deaths amongst this group were found to be significantly below the national average as a result of the 'healthy worker' effect—giving a standardized mortality rate (SMR) of 83%. The only SMR above 100% was for thyroid cancer based on just nine cases. However, when the incidence of disease was considered as a function of exposure, a more significant correlation with dose was found—that is the higher the overall dose received, the higher the risk of cancer, the mean value for the resulting risk estimates for leukaemia and for all malignant tumours being about double the current ICRP risk estimates.

14.3.6 Patients undergoing medical diagnosis with ionizing radiation

Patients exposed to ionizing radiation during medical examination have provided substantial evidence of carcinogenesis but even though the number of individuals is large, difficulties include the low doses received and hence low incidence rates of cancer, in the uncertainties in the dosimetry itself, and confounding factors such as the prevalence of pre-existing disease with poorer prognosis.

14.3.7 Patients treated with radiotherapy

There have been several studies on patients who have received radiotherapy, including those historically treated for non-malignant diseases, and therefore would have been expected to have a good prognosis and a normal expected lifetime. They provided strong evidence for the causal relationship between ionizing radiation and cancer; however, they still did not provide high-quality risk estimates. Even where there was good dosimetry and statistics, the fact that many of the patients received radiotherapy for pre-existing cancer made them a biased group which is unrepresentative of the normal population. Even where they were treated for non-malignant conditions, there remained a strong indication of bias, at least partially because of other existing comorbidities.

14.3.8 A-bomb survivors

Survivors of the atomic bombs dropped on Nagasaki and Hiroshima provide the most complete data and are still being studied extensively. There were about 120,000 residents in Hiroshima and Nagasaki in 1950 of whom about 94,000 were survivors following the atomic bombings of 1945. The rest were unexposed individuals. Sufficient dosimetric information could be estimated and/or calculated for about 76,000 survivors (1950) of whom just under 6,000 had died of cancer by 1985, on which the latest ICRP risk estimates are based. Of these a large proportion had cancers of types and at sites of the body showing a significant excess above expectation (e.g. leukaemia, malignant myeloma, colon, oesophagus, stomach, and lung).

However, interpretation of this data is complicated. First, the doses received by the exposed population leading to measurable increases in detected cancers are much greater (up to 1000 times or more) than those with which we are normally concerned in radiation protection. Secondly, many survivors were still alive at the conclusion of the study, and the manifestation of the consequences could not by definition be complete. Thirdly, the population on whom the bombs was dropped was different from those to which we wish to apply the data. There is strong evidence that susceptibility to cancer is affected by local considerations including environment and lifestyle, and being at war at that time, the normal sex and age population demographics were skewed because of the absence of men of military age. Finally, there were difficulties in the basic dosimetry—there were no radiation detectors that recorded the doses and dose rates experienced during the atomic bomb blasts, and the estimations and calculations have been subject to revaluations necessary to account for, *inter alia*, neutron shielding by buildings and absorption factors for the moisture in the air.

A further cohort of persons, mainly military personnel, witnessed atomic and nuclear bomb tests across the globe in the middle decades of the twentieth century, whose dosimetry records were finally released many years later, and provided further insight into the causal relationship between dose and risk of cancer.

14.4 **Framework for radiation protection**

Despite the deleterious effect discussed above, ionizing radiation has many potentially beneficial effects arising from its use, for example in medical practices. Radiation protection is concerned with obtaining those potential benefits whilst minimizing the costs of human exposure. The term **detriment** is used to define all deleterious effects, including not only the obvious health hazards but also incidental (monetary) costs associated with the mechanisms of establishing and implementing a practice using ionizing radiation and then the costs of interventions aimed at dose restriction.

Detriment may also be defined as a risk of harm to an individual, or as a collective risk to a population group. Even if both the individual risk and the size of the group are small, it may still be that harm is experienced by one or more individuals in the group, although it is of course unlikely. However, as either the individual risk or the size of the group increases, we may arrive at the situation where it is very likely that some individuals will suffer serious deleterious effects, but even so we will still not know who these individuals will be or even whether the harm is attributable to the ionizing radiation.

In 1977, the ICRP laid the current foundations for the framework of what is considered to be the modern era of radiation protection. Briefly, all human exposures to ionizing radiation should be governed by the following **principles:**

Justification—that no practice should be adopted unless its introduction produces a positive net benefit,

Optimization—all exposures should be kept **as low as reasonably practicable**, economic and social factors being taken into account (**ALARP**),

Limitation—doses to individuals (staff or the public) should not exceed appropriate limits.

Following the reassessment of risk estimates in 1990 and 2007, ICRP published revised recommendations. In 1990, the ICRP defined the concept of a network of the steps by which a group of individuals may be exposed to a specific source of ionizing radiation, whatever purpose is being made of it. This **Network** is defined as the chain of processes, or events and situations causing a human exposure to ionizing radiation. The **Source** is a term describing the item producing ionizing radiation. It will encompass the actual physical source, and could be a single radioactive source or X-ray machine, or a whole facility/establishment causing exposure (say) to the local population. The establishment will be carrying out a **Practice** (or series of Practices) such as diagnostic X-ray examinations which are the functions or activities increasing the overall exposure to ionizing radiation. Radiation protection then requires the Employer to consider **Interventions**—that is those activities which are designed to decrease the level of exposure received and the number of persons exposed.

In its 2007 review, ICRP drew distinctions in the way radiation protection should be considered for three types of exposure, occupational, medical, and public, in that they should be handled differently, being subject to different value judgements and practicable interventions. Furthermore ICRP also defined three exposure situations that may require different strategies to ensure that doses are reduced to as low as reasonably practicable, whilst still being subject to justification that the net benefit to exposed individuals or to society outweighs the risks. They are called Planned, Emergency, and Existing Situations.

Planned exposure situations describe those practices involving the use of ionizing radiation that can be fully planned in advance to ensure doses are optimized—for example setting up a radiology department as part of a newly built hospital. All the necessary structural shielding, layout, warns signs, interlocks, and protective equipment, etc. can be purchased and fitted/installed before the work with radiation begins for the first time.

Emergency situations require contingency plans to be operated, possibly allowing individuals to exceed normal dose limits if justified by resulting benefit. Therefore the statutory occupational dose limit of 20 mSv does not necessarily apply to emergency exposure situations. Furthermore, as a consequence of a radiological accident or incident, the public may also be exposed above the normal dose constraint or public dose limit, for instance due to having to eat contaminated foodstuffs. Whilst strategies may be adopted to reduce such exposures, it may not be possible to completely avoid increased public exposures because of such incidents.

Existing exposures describe situations such as radon in the home, occupational exposure to naturally occurring radioactive materials (NORM), or environmental contamination from previous operations, which were in existence before they were discovered by the authorities or a radiation employer. Strategies to reduce doses to optimized levels from such exposures may be prohibitively expensive and so the doses received occupationally or by the public may still be higher than might be expected from a fully pre-planned practice.

Before discussing the radiation protection legislation and the practical matters of implementing radiation protection measures in the Clinical Oncology setting, we shall define some radiation protection quantities and quantifying the risk of exposure to ionizing radiation as predicted by the data discussed previously.

14.5 **Radiation protection quantities and units**

Absorbed dose (measured in Gray, or milliGy (mGy) is considered appropriate for prescribing tumour doses because it relates to tissue reactions, however it does not relate directly to the probability of a stochastic effect. At the low doses encountered in occupational or public exposure to ionizing radiation, and for patients exposed for diagnostic purposes, it is necessary to introduce a dose quantity that will give an indication of this risk of harm. This requires taking into account the dose received, what type of radiation gave rise to the dose, and then to consider the tissues that have been irradiated and how sensitive those tissues are to radiation. The result of this process is to arrive at **effective dose**—the quantity defined by ICRP to give a measure of radiation risk.

14.5.1 **Equivalent dose and effective dose**

Some types of radiation potentially cause more damage to cells than others and are therefore riskier for the same absorbed dose: 1 mGy received from exposure to alpha particles is more likely to result in a cancer than the same absorbed dose from gamma rays. To take this into account, each type of radiation has been assigned a weighting factor. Multiplying the absorbed dose (Gy) by the radiation weighting factor gives a quantity called 'equivalent Dose', measured in Sievert (Sv). For photons (X-rays, gamma rays, and electrons or beta particles) the factor is 1, so that the equivalent dose is numerically equal to the absorbed dose. For other types of radiation, the weighting factors are greater (see Table 14.3). In effect, the weighting factor indicates how much more damaging the type of radiation is than X-rays. This can be written as an equation, where H is the equivalent dose, the product of D, the absorbed dose and W_R, the radiation weighting factor. Thus:

$$H = D \times W_R$$

Table 14.3 Radiation weighting factors

Radiation type	Weighting factor W_R
Photons: X- and gamma rays	1
Electrons	1
Neutrons	5–20, depending on energy
Alpha particles	20

If there is more than one type of radiation making up the exposure, the equivalent doses from each type are added together.

The weighting factor is based on a quantity called the 'relative biological effectiveness' (RBE) of the radiation, however it is not equal to the RBE. Weighting factors have been rounded to values such as 1, 10, and 20. For most of the radiation encountered in radiotherapy work (i.e. X-rays and electrons), the radiation weighting factor will be 1, so that the mean absorbed dose to a tissue and the equivalent dose will be numerically equal.

At this stage it is necessary also to consider the relative sensitivities of the tissues and organs being exposed to the ionizing radiation. These differences in such radiosensitivity are due to differences in the cellular replication rates for those tissues (faster replication rates implying a higher radiosensitivity), compounded by the fact that younger persons will also have more rapidly dividing cells in all tissues than older persons. This is then accounted for by applying a factor to represent the relative radiosensitivity of each tissue or organ—and that will be based on an estimate of the risk posed by the dose to the tissue.

Usually when a person is exposed to ionizing radiation, a part or the whole of the body is irradiated and a number of tissues receive some dose. To define the overall risk to a human exposed it is necessary to add up the contributions of doses received by each tissue/organ, adjusted for their relative radiosensitivity. This is taken into account by defining tissue weighting factors, whereby if the whole body and all tissues/organs were uniformly exposed then the individual weighting factors would all add up to 1. Thus for each tissue, the equivalent dose calculated above is multiplied by the tissue weighting factor and the 'effective dose' is worked out by adding together the contributions from all the tissues. If H_T is the equivalent dose to a tissue T and W_T is the tissue weighting factor for that tissue, the effective dose is defined by the following summation of the product of T and W_T for all the tissues exposed (the unit is still called the Sievert):

$$E = \Sigma\, H_T \times W_T$$

The tissue weighting factors were revised in 2007. The values are shown in Table 14.4. Note that:

- not all tissues are listed separately,
- there are only a few different values for weighting factors,
- several tissues have the same weighting factor.

Unlisted tissues are not immune to radiation but rather they have a lower sensitivity which only when considered collectively contributes in any significance to the effective dose. Calculating the effective dose using this methodology gives a sufficiently good estimate of risk to reflect present knowledge. For any practical situation, the estimate of the risk to a person exposed to radiation would not be improved by refining the tissue weighting factors further.

Calculating the effective dose results in a single number, whatever the pattern of radiation exposure over the body. This allows comparison of radiation doses from quite different types of exposure. For example, a frequently used comparison is that a

Table 14.4 Tissue weighting factors

Tissue	Weighting factor W_T
Gonads	0.08
Bone marrow (red)	0.12
Breast	0.12
Colon	0.12
Lung	0.12
Stomach	0.12
Bladder	0.04
Liver	0.04
Oesophagus	0.04
Thyroid	0.04
Bone surface	0.01
Brain	0.01
Salivary glands	0.01
Skin	0.01
Remainder	0.12
Total	**1**

chest X-ray gives about the same radiation dose as a return flight between the United Kingdom and Spain. Whether this reassures patients having X-rays or frightens holidaymakers is another question—the perception of risk is an important issue to consider when trying to convey the relative benefit and risk of a diagnostic test involving radiation exposure to get informed consent. A chest X-ray involves exposure of just part of the body to X-rays. A flight involves exposure of the whole body to enhanced levels of cosmic radiation, which is a mixture of gamma rays and various exotic types of high-energy ionizing particles. Nevertheless, the process of calculating effective dose results in a similar number for each exposure.

14.6 **Risk estimation and the dose response model**

Although many of the sources of data described in this chapter have led to a 'gold standard'—a clear understanding of quantifiable risk of ionizing radiation exposure causing harm in the form of cancer within a manageable level of uncertainty—the actual data are based on high dose exposures from about 0.5–4 Sv effective dose, and in many cases from doses received at very high dose rates. The problem for radiation protection is that most of the exposures that are of interest are much lower—of the order of a few mSv up to 20–30 mSv effective dose—and received

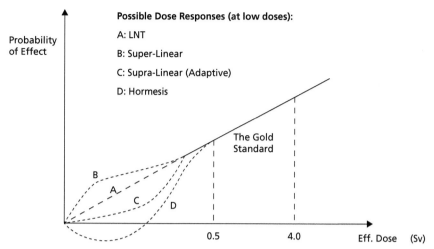

Figure 14.2 Possible response curves for radiation exposure at lower doses.

slowly over a much longer period. It is therefore necessary to consider how to ex-trapolate back from the gold standard to this lower dose/risk region of the curve (see Figure 14.2).

It might seem reasonable to assume a simply linear relationship and to extrapo-late back by drawing a straight line back to zero. This assumption is known as the 'linear no-threshold model' (LNT). However, when looking at a variety of epidemio-logical *and in-vitro* cellular studies of the dose/response relationship at lower doses, there are a number of conflicting results and subsequent conjectures as to the reasons why they may be different to the LNT. Some data suggest that cells are proportionally more sensitive to radiation carcinogenesis at lower doses than the LNT model would predict, and other data suggest not only are cells more resistive (adaptive) to such damage at lower doses but that radiation exposure at low levels may indeed even lead to a hormetic—beneficial—effect in providing a protection against subsequent cellular exposure to radiation or other carcinogenetic factors such as pollution, etc. In other words that a little bit of radiation may do good rather than harm. These competing responses are represented in Figure 14.2.

Given the confounding factors that might be increasing the uncertainties at lower doses, and the overall statistical uncertainties, ICRP suggests the best model for the purposes of managing radiation protection in the workplace and for the public is the LNT model. It is the most straightforward to implement, steering a middle course be-tween the extremes of the observed data.

With an assumed linear response of the cancer risk to radiation dose received, it is then possible to quantify it—and the data suggest that it is about **5% per Sievert** for fatal cancers (or **0.005% per mSv**)—that is for every 100 healthy adult persons in a cohort exposed to 1 Sv effective dose (or 100,000 exposed to 1 mSv), it would be ex-pected that five excess fatal cancers would develop in that cohort. This of course is an

Table 14.5 Risk figures for fatal cancer against age at exposure in % per Sv

Age at Exposure:	Male:	Female:	Average:
0	13	16	14.5
5	14	17	15.5
10	13	16	14.5
15	11	15	13.0
20	9.2	11	10.1
30	5.8	6.4	6.1
40	4.8	5.1	4.95
50	4.7	4.7	4.7
60	3.9	3.7	3.8
70	2.1	2.1	2.1
80	0.88	0.89	0.89

indicative figure, and there would be no way to predict *which* five persons for every 100 (or 100,000) in the cohort would be the ones to suffer the harm.

It is useful at this point to also consider again the delay—the latency period from initiating event (the exposure) to the progression of a cancer to its final consequence; for leukaemias it might be from 2 to 10 years, and for solid tumours from 5 to 30+ years. This delay has a potentially significant effect on the risks suffered by cohorts of persons across the full age range in a population. Furthermore there are inherent differences in cellular sensitivity to radiation between young and old, and between males and females. This has been studied extensively and has led ICRP to publish age- and sex-related risk figures, as summarized in Table 14.5.

As can be seen from Table 14.5, children less than 10 years old are up to three times more likely to have a fatal cancer induced by radiation exposure than a middle-aged adult, and persons older than around 80 years old are less than a fifth as likely compared to the middle-aged adult. This of course is of potential significance and importance for the process of justification in the deliberate medical exposures of patients, as examinations to children with higher risks will require higher perceived benefits to merit proceeding. Those on much older patients, whilst not being trivialized, may not warrant such close attention.

14.7 **Summary of legislative requirements**

14.7.1 **The Ionising Radiations Regulations 2017 (IRR17)**

As discussed earlier, legislation in radiation protection is principally determined by the recommendations of the ICRP. Over the decades more information on radiation risks has been gathered and analysed and this has led to the most recent updated recommendations published in 2007.

Health and safety legislation in Europe is developed primarily by the European Community (EC) through European Directives. In 2013 the EC published a revised Basic Safety Standards (BSS) Directive (2013/59/EURATOM) based on the recommendations of ICRP Report 103. This Directive required implementation by member states in their national legislative framework before 6 February 2018. The Ionising Radiation Regulations 2017 (IRR17) was a major piece of legislation which implemented the non-medical aspects of the BSS Directive in the UK. IRR17 is a Statutory Instrument—a set of regulations made under an enabling Act of Parliament, and as with all hazards in the workplace this is the Health and Safety at Work Act 1974.

The three basic ICRP principles of radiation protection—*justification*, *optimization*, and *limitation*—are to be met through compliance with IRR17, and as with all hazards in the workplace covered by the various regulations under the Act, the Employer is recognized as being ultimately responsible for the safety of staff, visitors to the workplace (including patients) and the public from the ionizing radiation being used. This is primarily expected to be achieved through first justifying the need to use ionizing radiations with consequent occupational exposure (quite straightforward for medical uses), then providing a governance and management structure for ionizing radiation safety (within general health and safety governance and oversight). The Employer will also be expected to appoint a registered radiation protection adviser (RPA) to provide appropriate information, instructions and training to all staff who work directly or indirectly with the radiation.

The employer is expected to carry out prior radiation risk assessments to determine the level of magnitude of the hazards and risks posed by each source of ionizing radiation. As a result, and according to the level of hazard and risk present, areas where the work with ionizing radiation is carried out will require designation; the most significant hazard/risks areas being designated as Controlled Areas, for example a radiotherapy treatment room. An area must be classed as Controlled if it is likely that an individual may receive an effective dose of more than 6 mSv per year. There is also a lower level of designation where doses received, although not currently of concern, could change and become significant over time if not kept under review—these areas being called Supervised Areas, such as a radiotherapy treatment unit control area. An area is designated as Supervised if an individual is likely to receive an effective dose of more than 1 mSv per year. All other areas in or adjacent to the workplace may be deemed to be such a low hazard as to be viewed as public, or unrestricted. The purpose of area designation is to ensure that no person may receive more than the statutory dose limits (see below). The Employer must ensure that all designated areas are adequately demarcated so that staff and other persons may recognize the hazard present, and that Local Rules are available—a document to summarize the information and instructions required to be followed by all persons entering designated areas to ensure their safety. To further ensure that the Local Rules are followed by all staff, it is expected that the Employer appoint a radiation protection supervisor (RPS) for the work in each area of the facility.

The dose limits specified in IRR17 are summarized in Table 14.6. These are based on the internationally recognized limit of what is considered acceptable annual risk of death arising from occupational hazards—that a worker should not be exposed to an

Table 14.6 Annual dose limits in IRR17 (mSv)

	Employees		Public
	> 18 years old	Trainees under 18	and all persons under 16 years
Effective Dose	20 (or 100 in 5 years)	6	1
Equivalent Doses:	20	15	15
Lens of eye	500	150	50
Skin*	500	150	50
Other tissue/organ			

(*—Skin dose averaged over 1 cm² of skin)

annual risk of death from any occupational hazard of more than 1 in 1000. As the risk of developing cancer quoted above of 5% per Sievert, 20 mSv is equivalent to 0.1%—1 in 1000—and is thus the effective dose limit for workers. The public dose limit is based again on an internationally recognized premise that the public, including the most vulnerable members (the young and the unwell) should not be exposed on average to a risk of more than the order of 1 in 100,000. Given that the vast majority of members of the public are not exposed to radiation at all as a consequence of the work activities carried out by any single employer, a dose limit of 1 mSv (equivalent to 1 in 20,000 risk) seems reasonable.

The dose limits specified in terms of equivalent doses for different organs or tissues are based on ensuring that they do not receive a dose more than the threshold dose for those tissues—to avoid the possibility of deterministic tissue reactions.

There will be some staff who, due to the nature of the particular tasks they perform and the way they have to be done, and as a result of the risk assessments might be expected to receive a more significant proportion (normally three-tenths) of a dose limit. Those workers are expected to be formally designated as Classified Workers, and will have to be issued with personal radiation monitors (thermoluminescent dosimeters (TLD) (see section 5.6.1.1) or similar) so that particular attention can be given to the doses they receive, and follow-up annual medicals can confirm that they are fit to continue the work with ionizing radiation. Other staff may receive lower but still measurable doses and it will be decided as a result of a risk assessment that they should also be monitored, although it will be expected that they will not ordinarily receive doses that will be a cause of concern.

Irrespective of whether systems have been put in place to ensure that staff or the public will receive doses lower than the limits, the Employer is expected to go further to ensure that the actual occupational and public doses received are indeed minimized. Specifically, it is not sufficient merely to meet the dose limits. Employers should take steps, if possible, to reduce exposure to dose further. In doing so they are allowed to consider the social and economic factors, including the costs of interventions towards dose reduction. This achieves optimization—that doses are as low as *reasonably practicable*.

14.7.2 The Ionising Radiation (Medical Exposures) Regulations 2017 (IR(ME)R)

These regulations can be seen primarily as ensuring that the Employer establishes a framework for achieving justification and optimization for every patient's medical exposure to ionizing radiation. It should be noted that there can be no dose limitation applied to medical exposures—any restriction on patients having a diagnostic or therapeutic medical procedure simply because they had had previous exposures leading to some arbitrary dose limit would be inappropriate. So medical exposures must be justified on an individual case basis, and the dose delivered then tailored to achieve the clinical need—that is either minimized whilst getting adequate diagnostic information, or planned and delivered to achieve the therapeutic aim (treating a cancer).

The regulations are enforced by the Care Quality Commission (CQC) on behalf of the Department of Health and Social Care, and they set out the roles and legal responsibilities for certain defined individuals—not just the Employer but the Referrer, the Practitioner, the Operator, and the Medical Physics Expert. These are roles crucial to patient radiation safety. A person may have more than one of these roles during a patient's journey.

The **Referrer** examines a patient who appears to be suffering from a clinical condition and thinks that the patient may benefit from a medical exposure, whether for confirmation of the diagnosis of the condition or for its treatment. They refer that patient on to an appropriate specialist who can determine whether to go ahead with the diagnostic test or the treatment. The referral contains appropriate information about the patient and the suspected clinical condition, and the legal responsibility for including that information in the referral remains with the Referrer. Usually the Referrer is a doctor or dentist, however non-medical referrers are allowed under the Regulations, given appropriate training.

The **Practitioner** is the specialist in using radiation to diagnose, or guide, or treat clinical conditions. That person will have the in-depth knowledge to be able to ascertain whether the procedure suggested by the referral is indeed appropriate for the patient and that they will thus benefit from it, that is the Practitioner determines whether the medical radiation exposure is *justified*. The Practitioner will then authorize the exposure to proceed, and they or the Operator will be expected to write a report to the Referrer giving the results of the procedure, to confirm diagnosis or that treatment was completed successfully.

The **Operator** is any member of staff who is trained and entitled according to departmental procedures to carry out practical tasks relating to radiotherapy or related imaging radiation exposures. Operator tasks can include contouring, planning, and checking a treatment plan; operating treatment and imaging equipment; quality assurance of radiation equipment; and clinical patient review. Operator tasks may be carried out by oncologists, therapy radiographers, clinical scientists, and technologists.

Furthermore, in the absence of the Practitioner, the Operator may be permitted to authorize patient exposures. Examples of this are authorizing additional imaging (e.g. CBCT), therapy radiographer authorization of palliative treatment exposures and physics' authorization of treatment plans for sites such as breast or prostate.

Such authorization to act in that way can only be given to the Operator by a Practitioner who must set out clearly in writing the scope or range of exposures, the clinical conditions, and the criteria for which the Operator can make the decision to proceed.

Note that a clinical oncologist can therefore be a referrer, practitioner, and operator. The **Medical Physics Expert** (MPE) has responsibility for several matters set out specifically in the Regulations with the broad objective to ensure that the Employer understands the requirements for compliance with the law, and that patients receive optimized medical radiation treatment and imaging on appropriate equipment which is operating safely.

The MPE will be involved in range of matters including advising on dosimetry and quality assurance, carrying out physical measurements for the evaluation of patient doses delivered, the optimization of treatment planning, and dose delivery. As required, the MPE will be involved in the preparation of technical specifications for new equipment and installation design, followed by carrying out acceptance testing of the new equipment, and then defining and performing a schedule of routine quality assurance testing, including surveillance of the safety aspects.

14.7.2.1 ARSAC

IR(ME)R specifically requires that all administrations of medicinal radioactive substances (radiopharmaceuticals) whether for diagnostic imaging or other testing, or for treatment (radionuclide therapies) must be carried out under the direction of licensed clinicians (as Practitioners) using appropriately licensed facilities. Practitioner licences are issued on application to qualified and experienced clinicians by the Secretary of State for Health after advice from the Administration of Radioactive Substances Advisory Committee (ARSAC) that considers each application. ARSAC also receives applications from employers for licensing hospitals with suitable facilities, equipment, and staff resources, including support from suitably qualified medical physicists and clinical technologists, to carry out such diagnostic and therapeutic procedures involving radioactive substances on their premises.

14.7.2.2 Unintended or accidental exposures

Human error and the possibility of equipment faults leading to unintended or accidental exposures cannot be completely eliminated, so that when such incidents do occur, an investigation and root cause analysis of events must be carried out. Such an investigation will involve the clinician responsible for the patient's care, the staff involved in the incident, and the MPE/RPA to carry out an assessment of the significance of the dose received because of the incident in relation to the intended dose.

The regulations require that any incidents involving more significant unintended or accidental exposure of patients are formally reported to CQC as the enforcing authority. In this context 'significant' can be defined as a received exposure due to the incident which is at a level where the future clinical management and treatment of the patient may be affected. These incidents include where the wrong patient has been exposed, the right patient has received an exposure to the wrong part of the body (a geographical miss), or a process failure has led to significant over- or underexposure. The CQC has published guidance on how to determine whether reporting is required. The factors that should be used in determining whether an incident is reportable are given in Table 14.7. Note that an 'Accidental exposure' occurs when an

Table 14.7 Criteria for deciding whether an incident is reportable to CQC under IR(ME)R

Notification code	Exposure category	Criteria for notification
Accidental exposure:		
1 (England only)	All modalities including therapy	3 mSv effective dose or above (adult) 1 mSv effective dose or above (child)
1 (Northern Ireland & Scotland)	All modalities including therapy	All, regardless of dose
Unintended exposure:		
All modalities including nuclear medicine and radiotherapy pre-treatment imaging		
2.1	Intended dose less than 0.3 mSv	3 mSv or above (adult) 1 mSv or above (child)
2.2	Intended dose between 0.3 mSv and 2.5 mSv	10 or more times than intended
2.3	Intended dose between 2.5 mSv and 10 mSv	25 mSv or above
2.4	Intended dose more than 10mSv	2.5 or more times than intended
4.1	Radiotherapy pre-treatment planning scans	If CT planning scan needs to be repeated twice to obtain an appropriate dataset (three scans in total, including the intended scan)
4.2	Radiotherapy treatment verification images	Set-up error leads to three or more imaging exposures in a single fraction (including the intended image, i.e. three images in total) OR when the number of additional imaging exposures is 20% greater than intended over the course of treatment or than was described in the protocol
5	Foetal All modalities	Where there has been a failure in the procedure for making pregnancy enquiries, AND the resultant foetal dose is 1 mGy or more
Radiotherapy delivered dose (including brachytherapy)		
7.1	Therapy over-exposure	Delivered dose to the planned treatment volume (PTV) and/or organs at risk (OAR) is 1.1 or more times (whole course) or 1.2 or more times (any fraction) the intended dose
7.2	Therapy under-exposure	Delivered dose to the PTV is 0.9 or less times the intended dose (whole course)

(continued)

Table 14.7 Continued

Notification code	Exposure category	Criteria for notification
Radiotherapy geographical miss (including brachytherapy)		
8.1	Total	All total geographical misses, even for a single fraction or significant part thereof
8.2	Partial	Where the miss exceeds 2.5 times the locally defined error margin AND the guideline dose factors above (as 7.1 & 7.2) for the PTV or OAR are exceeded
Nuclear medicine therapy		
9.1	Selective Internal Radiation Therapy	Delivered activity is outside +/−20% of the prescribed activity.
9.2	All other nuclear medicine therapies	Delivered activity is outside +/−10% of the prescribed activity.
Complementary notification codes		
M	More than one individual exposed within the same incident/theme. (suffix with number code as above)	All cases regardless of dose
E	Equipment fault exposure (suffix as above)	
V	Voluntary notification (suffix as above)	
C	Clinically significant event (suffix as above)	

individual receives an exposure when *none* was intended. An 'Unintended Exposure' occurs when an individual receives an exposure that was significantly greater or less than intended. When Unintended Exposures occur, they are often due to procedural or human error but those including equipment malfunction should also be reported.

The multiplication factor to be used is defined as the total dose from the incident divided by the dose from the intended exposure alone.

CQC suggests that employers should also consider reporting incidents which do not meet the criteria for compulsory notification, hence the inclusion of code V for voluntary reporting. The CQC is clear that all incidents as well as near misses, no matter how insignificant, should be thoroughly investigated by the Employer to determine the root causes and the corrective actions designed to avoid recurrence. All persons involved in the care of the patient, and specifically the procedure during which an incident occurred, should also be involved in the investigation.

14.7.3 The Environmental Permitting Regulations 2016

The Environmental Permitting Regulations (EPR) are designed to protect staff and the public from the hazards and risk arising from the use of a wide range of potentially toxic substances, including radioactive substances. This is primarily achieved by requiring the employer to ensure that the amounts of radioactive substances held and used are controlled, and that any waste arising from that use is accumulated and then disposed of responsibly. All of this must be done within defined limits and conditions set out on permits issued by the Environment Agencies (for England and the devolved administrations) under the regulations. Schedule 23 of EPR is the section specifically devoted to the particular requirements for using and disposing of radioactive substances, including for medical purposes.

In applying for a permit to hold, use, and dispose of radioactive substances, the employer must compare the necessity to use radioactivity to the availability, appropriateness and cost of any other alternatives—called a Best Available Techniques analysis—and to then carry out a Radiological Hazard Assessment of the resulting waste discharges to the environment in terms of the radiation doses to humans and to other species that might be received.

The regulations cover all uses of radioactive substances across all sectors including the range of medical uses in hospitals, both unsealed (liquid, vapour, or gas) and sealed (solid, encapsulated), and including High-Activity Sealed Sources (HASS). These HASS are the sources found in high dose-rate (HDR) brachytherapy machines (amongst other uses), and which in themselves present a significant hazard to anyone directly exposed to them for a period of time.

However, most of EPR2016 is not focused on radiation safety *per se*, but on the impact of uncontrolled discharges of radioactivity to the environment potentially affecting the public and non-human species. One other aspect of the regulations specific to HASS, and other sources that may be of significant hazard, is that there needs to be in place a regimen of physical and information security measures around the storage and use of such sources, so that they cannot be accessed by any person unauthorized to do so. Furthermore, they must be disposed of either by agreement to be returned to the manufacturer/supplier, or to a contractor approved and licensed to recycle or dispose of them in the appropriate way.

14.8 **Practical radiation protection—design and management of RT facilities**

Radiation protection measures can and should be built into the facility at the design stage. It should be possible for the facility to be fully planned with radiation safety in mind—in the terminology of ICRP it is a Planned Exposure Situation—which allows for little compromise and maximized safety.

The design of the facility will be based on three practical aspects:

◆ The use of shielding to avoid significant exposure to any person;

◆ The use of increased distance between the source and any persons to reduce the dose rates from any exposures;

◆ Minimizing the time during which any person is directly exposed to the ionizing radiation.

For most of the work of a Radiotherapy department, reducing the time of exposure, or using distance as a means to protect persons from the radiation sources, are not feasible ways of achieving ALARP doses to staff and the public. That leaves only the first measure—shielding—as the chief way of ensuring safety in such a facility. So let us look at a generic design for the treatment room, and then highlight some specific features which will be common to all types of treatment modality and those which will be more specific in different modalities.

For external beam therapies that are electrically produced—that is using linear accelerators (linacs)—the radiation hazard has several components:

- the primary beam
- secondary scatter from—
  - the patient
  - the walls
  - any equipment in the room
- radiation leakage from the treatment head

The facility must have enough shielding present in the walls, ceiling, and floor to reduce all these contributions to acceptable dose rates outside the facility. Tomotherapy systems (see section 11.6.2) use the same geometry as a CT scanner and have an intrinsic primary beam stopper to absorb the beam exiting from the

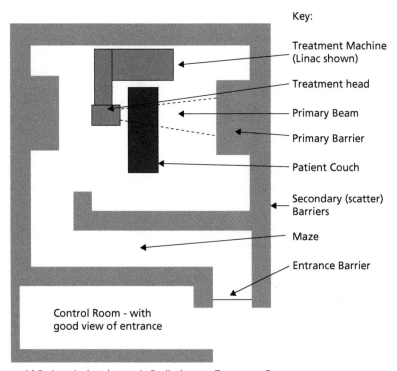

Figure 14.3 A typical and generic Radiotherapy Treatment Room.

patient such that the walls, floor, and ceiling of the treatment room do not require a primary barrier. Conversely, CyberKnife® systems (see section 11.6.1) are a linear accelerator on the head of a robotic arm that can point in nearly any direction around the patient and therefore all walls and the floor must then be primary barriers.

For systems using HASS for HDR brachytherapy, the source itself when driven out from its container into the patient produces a primary radiation field in practically all directions which is then absorbed and scattered by the patient, walls, and equipment within the room. Again, the walls, ceiling, and floor must have sufficient shielding to reduce the dose rates outside to acceptable levels. The room will also require the physical security measures previously mentioned to meet the requirements for preventing access to the HASS by unauthorized persons.

Such facilities may or may not make use of an entrance maze (see Figure 14.3) to avoid the requirement for a heavily shielded door which would require an electromechanical drive. The maze would have to be designed such that the radiation scattered along it has been reduced in intensity to the extent that the dose rate at the entrance is at acceptable levels.

For all these facilities, one of the major risks is that a person other than the patient may remain inside the facility whilst the treatment is initiated, or may enter accidentally during the middle of a treatment. It is essential that systems are in place that ensure the patient is the only person in the room before the treatment begins:

◆ the last person to leave the room before the treatment checks that no-one else remains in the room (other than the patient!), presses a button to confirm, then presses another in the control room to verify—only then will the equipment allow the treatment to be started.

◆ CCTV should be available so that the operator is able always to see inside the room during the treatment.

◆ there should be a barrier at the entrance, with interlocks installed which will trip if anyone enters, terminating the treatment. If there is a well-designed maze, the barrier will not require shielding, so can be a door, a gate, or even a light beam. The room will also have hazard warning signs and lights as discussed earlier in this chapter and as required by the regulations.

Only facilities where low dose rate (LDR) implants are carried out (e.g. iodine seeds for prostate brachytherapy, section 12.3.3.2) do not depend on shielding as the primary measure for safety. The very low energy X-rays emitted from the seeds present a low hazard to staff whilst they are placed through an appropriately designed and shielded delivery system. Therefore, this can be carried out in a normal theatre facility without specialized shielding. Once the patient has been treated and discharged from hospital to return home with the seeds remaining in situ, they present a negligible hazard to persons standing more than 30–50 cm away. However, the patient should avoid prolonged close contact to reduce the risk to family and friends, and particularly to younger children.

14.9 **Summary**

Human exposure to ionizing radiation has the potential to cause harm, whether inducing immediate acute effects or by raising the risk of developing cancer later in life. This knowledge has resulted from studies of people exposed to a range of radiation sources, and attempts have been made to understand the physical, chemical, and biological mechanisms for the damage and harm caused, to model the response of the cells and tissues, and to quantify that harm or risk of harm in relation to the radiation doses received.

Conversely, using ionizing radiation in medicine, both to diagnose and to treat patients, is considered justified in that the benefits to the patients are perceived to outweigh the risk of harm. The purpose of radiation protection in the hospital setting is to establish a management framework such that the patient receives radiation exposure to maximize the benefit whilst minimizing the risks, and to protect staff and any other persons so that they are not exposed to unacceptable radiation doses from those medical procedures.

Chapter 15

Quality in radiotherapy

Andrew Morgan and Niall MacDougall

15.1 Introduction

A quotation often attributed to American industrialist and car manufacturer Henry Ford states: 'Quality means doing it right when no-one is watching.'

Quality can be a difficult term to define. The definition can depend on the circumstances to which it is applied. Dictionary definitions of quality include 'of a high standard' or 'a feature of something that makes it different from something else'.

Members of a radiotherapy multidisciplinary team (MDT) would probably state that maximizing favourable patient outcomes by defining target volumes correctly, delivering the treatment as accurately as possible, and correct calibration of the treatment machines represent quality.

Patients' perspectives on the quality of their radiotherapy are likely to be more experiential, such as how long they had to wait for their treatment, how comfortable were the chairs in the waiting area, and how long would it be before someone removes that dead fish from the tank in reception.

15.2 Quality

Quality underpins all modern radiotherapy processes, for good reasons that we'll discuss in this chapter. We will start with definitions of some key terms which will recur in this chapter and introductory explanations.

Quality: The standard of something as measured against other things of a similar kind.

15.2.1 Quality Management System (QMS)

Generically, a QMS is comprised of the procedures, policies, and processes to enable an organization to deliver its essential business to meet customer requirements. In the case of radiotherapy, the customer is the patient.

15.2.2 QMS in radiotherapy

Following a high-profile UK radiotherapy incident in 1988, the Department of Health (DoH) encouraged all radiotherapy centres to establish and maintain a QMS.

In 2008, the multi-professional report 'Towards Safer Radiotherapy' (TSRT) recommended that every department should have a 'fully funded, externally accredited quality management system in place'. Accredited in this case means that an independent body has determined through inspection that the QMS meets the requirements of a recognized quality standard, in this case BS ENISO 9001:2000. This standard has since developed further to ISO 9001:2015

15.2.3 Quality assurance (QA) and quality control (QC)

Two terms (occasionally used interchangeably) are **quality assurance** (QA) and **quality control** (QC). They are certainly closely linked but subtlety different.

Quality assurance covers all procedures that ensure the safe delivery of the radiotherapy prescription, optimizing dose to the target volume and minimizing dose to normal tissue. QA in radiotherapy involves all aspects of the radiotherapy process, with cooperative contributions from all relevant staff groups.

Quality control is the term applied to the specific measurements and tests undertaken to ensure that the standards specified in the QMS are maintained. In the case of linear accelerators for example, QC checks assure that the equipment performs to the same level as when the equipment was first commissioned. If not, QC results can inform the changes required to restore equipment performance to the required level.

It is hopefully self-evident that a culture of high quality will result in radiotherapy delivery that is safe, accurate, and precise.

15.3 Accuracy and precision

Accuracy and precision are two words which are again often used interchangeably. However, in scientific terms each has a specific and independent meaning. A measurement can be highly accurate but not precise or any combination of high/low accuracy and high/low precision, which may not make too much sense at first. Note that precision is another term for reproducibility.

Figure 15.1a shows four possible combinations for accuracy and precision. In this case, the example is of 12 arrows fired at a target, aiming to hit the triangle in the middle. Precision is a measure of how closely the arrows are grouped on the target. Accuracy is how close the whole group of arrows is to the centre of the target.

From this arrow/target analogy, we can see it's not possible to determine accuracy from one arrow unless one has knowledge of the precision of the person firing the arrows.

All measurement techniques require their accuracy and precision quantifying before one can rely on individual measurements. This is the case for many examples in this book.

15.3.1 The clinical implications of the accuracy and precision of radiotherapy delivery

Figure 15.1b shows the relationship between absorbed dose and tumour control probability (TCP) and normal tissue complication probability (NTCP). These graphs are

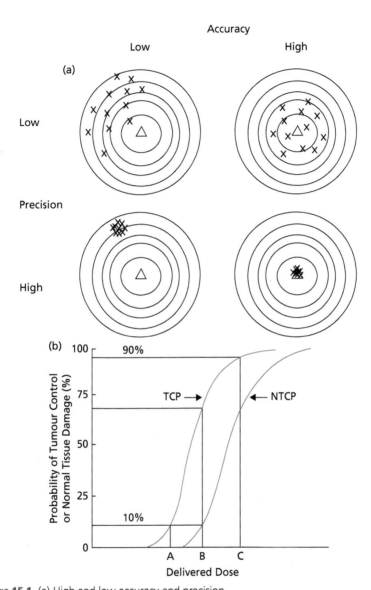

Figure 15.1 (a) High and low accuracy and precision.
(b) Changes of TCP and NTCP with dose.
Reproduced from http://indico.ictp.it/event/7955/session/0/contribution/1/material/slides/0.ppt

theoretical and depend on multiple factors. However, they demonstrate the need for accurate and precise radiation dosimetry.

The graph shows that delivery of dose A results in no NTCP but a TCP of only 10%. For a larger number of patients to have their tumour controlled, the dose must be increased.

- Dose B will result in a TCP of around 70% and an NTCP of 10%. The gradients of both the TCP and NTCP curves are quite steep and hence the likely outcome for the patient will be significantly influenced by small changes in dose.
- If the dose is greater than B, the TCP will increase which is a good thing. However, the NTCP will also increase, which is not so good.
- If the dose is less than B then the NTCP will decrease, but the TCP will also decrease.
- Dose C results in the highest TCP, but also the highest NTCP and is likely to be unacceptable clinically.

An assumption in this example is that the tumour is uniformly irradiated. In cases where the tumour may be partially missed by the radiation beams (often termed a 'geographic' miss) the lower delivered dose reduces the TCP, which increases the risk of a poor patient outcome.

The steps required to ensure accuracy and precision in radiotherapy will be discussed later in this chapter.

15.4 **Quality control checks in radiotherapy**

15.4.1 **Treatment equipment QC**

The range of complex equipment available in a radiotherapy department has grown rapidly over the past twenty years and a significant part of the work of a radiotherapy physics service is spent undertaking quality control checks and interpreting the results. Guidance on such checks is provided by professional bodies. In the United Kingdom, the relevant professional body is the Institute of Physics and Engineering in Medicine (IPEM). Report 81 (2nd edition) provides QC guidance on all equipment—imaging, planning, treatment, and dosimetry—with details on check methodologies, frequencies, and tolerances. Table 15.1 shows a representative selection of checks expected to be carried out on linear accelerators. It is by no means comprehensive. Note that two tolerances are usually applied to QC checks. The lower limit is called the Action Limit. Any performance deviations exceeding this level require further action investigation by a competent individual, but the clinical service may continue. There is also a second tolerance, the Suspension Limit, beyond which the equipment must be removed from clinical use for remedial works. Suggested Action Limits are shown in Table 15.1.

Daily QC is often performed by treatment radiographers with other checks being undertaken by dosimetrists, physicists, or linear accelerator (linac) engineers.

QC checks specific to brachytherapy are discussed in section 12.7. However they are determined, parameters related to radiation beam performance are always compared to the benchmark data acquired during the period of machine commissioning (section 11.8.3) before it enters clinical use.

15.4.2 **Treatment plan checking QC**

The pre-treatment and treatment planning processes can be complex. There are several interfaces where key information is passed between various staff groups. Any mistakes

Table 15.1 Suggested action limits

Test and frequency	Action limit
Daily	
Quick output check with simple dosemeter	+/–3%
Light field size for a 10 × 10 cm field	2 mm
Crosswire and isocentric laser coincidence	2 mm
Optical Distance Indicator compared to lasers	2 mm
Weekly	
Output constancy check with independent dosemeter	+/–3%
Monthly	
Emergency Power Off Switches	Functional
Gantry and collimator rotation scale accuracy	+/–0.5°
Distance indication at different FSDs	2 mm
Output calibration check using calibrated ion chambers	+/–2%
Three monthly	
Dose output variation with gantry angle	+/–2%
Six monthly	
Dose output variation with dose rate	1%
Annually	
Beam flatness and symmetry checks at all gantry angles	Flatness and symmetry both within +/–2% of reference values
Couch deflection under simulated patient load	5 mm
Definitive check on isocentre diameter	2 mm

introduced at this stage have the potential to go undetected and may result in a treatment error.

After they have been produced and approved, all plans should undergo a rigorous check of all parameters before they are used for treatment. This 'plan check' needs to be undertaken by someone who has been fully independent of the plan production process. Checking regimes will generally include patient identification, laterality, target definition including application of margins, choice of modality/energy, dose distribution including adequacy of coverage of targets and of sparing of organs at risk (OARs). A plan Monitor Unit (MU) check will take place at this point in the pathway. This is usually done using a software package which is completely independent from the system used to produce the plan. It can accept patient contour data from the main planning system but uses a different dose calculation method to determine the dose to the patient if the TPS MU were applied.

15.4.3 Treatment plan verification

While an independent MU check can provide some confidence in the veracity of a relatively simple, non-modulated treatment plan, the complexity of some treatment techniques such as volumetric modulated arc therapy (VMAT) make some users uncomfortable with the concept of relying solely on a second calculation to demonstrate the correctness of the delivered dose. There are several safety options available.

15.4.3.1 Direct treatment measurement

Several phantom devices are commercially available, containing a large number of detectors (usually silicon diodes, see section 5.6.1.2) in either planar or cylindrical arrays. These devices can be placed on the treatment couch and exposed to the treatment beams for a given patient. The doses measured by the diodes can be compared to those calculated by the treatment planning system (TPS) in the phantom.

15.4.3.2 EPID base dosimetry

The electronic portal imager (EPID, see section 11.3.7.1) on the linac can be used to measure the radiation beam from the treatment plan and be compared to predicted doses from either the TPS or the secondary MU check software.

15.4.3.3 Comparing dose distributions—the Gamma Index

When using VMAT/intensity modulated radiotherapy (IMRT) it is likely that steep dose gradients will be present. It is possible that at a point in or close to a steep dose gradient, there will be a large dose difference between measured and calculated doses. This may not be as significant as it sounds if the point is within a small distance, say 2–3 mm of the correct dose. This is the basis for what is known as the gamma index, a parameter used to assess the quality of highly modulated plans. The gamma index combines a check of positional accuracy and dose accuracy to give a single number answer at all points in the distribution, if the values are between 0 and 1 then the delivery is acceptable within the dose percentage and millimetre distance to agreement limits you have set. A typical gamma index may be based a dose tolerance of 3% and a geometric tolerance of 2 mm. Pass rates are usually agreed locally but are often in the range 95–98% as a minimum.

15.4.4 *In-vivo* dosimetry

The next check, after confirming that the treatment plan is as intended, is checking that the treatment is delivered to the patient as intended. *In-vivo* dosimetry (IVD) is the measurement of the dose received by a patient during radiotherapy. In the wake of two radiotherapy incidents in the 2000s, the Chief Medical Officer's 2006 report covered the topic of safety in radiotherapy and recommended the routine use of IVD to reduce the risk of such events in future. The report re-ignited discussion within the United Kingdom on the cost effectiveness of IVD, the limited technology available in 2008 meant high staff time commitment was required. It was feared that allocating resources to the implementation and maintenance of IVD might result in errors elsewhere in the system.

15.4.4.1 On-skin detectors

A small detector—such as a silicon diode, thermoluminescent dosimeter (TLD), or metal oxide semiconductor field effect transistor (MOSFET) (see Chapter 5)—is positioned on the patient's skin within each radiation field before the start of the treatment exposure. The dose received is measured and compared with the value expected which has been calculated independently. This all sounds relatively straightforward but in practice, is far from it. Accurate diode measurements require multiple correction factors to account for beam energy, source-to-surface distance (SSD), temperature, field size, and oblique incidence. TLDs require processing post exposure and cannot provide a real-time read out of dose delivered. It is a very manual and imperfect process which fuelled the objections to IVD. While the arguments on the pros and cons of IVD rumbled on, treatment delivery technology advanced rapidly and from 2013 onwards the use of IMRT and VMAT increased significantly. Even the staunchest advocates of IVD would agree that point dose measurements would only be of use in a relatively uniform radiation field. In IMRT/VMAT, the dose is likely to vary significantly across the beam and measurements, making a single point dose measurement somewhat meaningless.

15.4.4.2 EPID and log file dosimetry

The IVD debate is being settled now with the advent of EPIDs (section 11.3.7.1) and log file based *in-vivo* dosimetry. These processes can be automated and use that day's patient cone beam computed tomography (CBCT) to give an anatomical representation of the dose delivered to the patient on every fraction. Log files are generated automatically by the linac to aid engineers to fault find. They contain records of the physical location of multileaf collimator (MLC) leaves (and many other things), the IVD systems can use this positional information to change the delivered dose to more agree with the actual (or what the log files report) MLC positions during treatment. If you would rather have an IVD system that measures dose, then there are systems that use EPIDs to directly measure dose received by the patient. An EPID is a silicon panel (Figure 11.10) mounted on the accelerator gantry, which unfolds opposite the treatment head. It detects the patient attenuated MV treatment beam and produces a 2D image of the treatment field, generating a greyscale map of the exit dose from the patient. These dose maps can then 'back projected' into the patient's CBCT and the actual delivered dose calculated, in a process akin to that described in section 8.3.1. So the EPID is continually capturing discrete frames of dose and a 3D dose map of the treatment is produced, for comparison with the treatment plan in 3D, using the gamma index as described above.

15.4.5 **Geometric verification of treatment delivery**

The accurate and precise delivery of radiotherapy is achieved by performing an imaging procedure immediately prior to treatment delivery. This process has been termed both image verification and image guidance, though the latter is now more commonly used.

Linacs are fitted with at least one type of imaging equipment (see sections 10.2 and 11.3.7). Initially, images were obtained using an EPID, such images could then be compared to a digitally reconstructed radiograph (DRR), generated from the planning CT dataset by treatment planning systems (TPS). Through most of the 1990s into the 2000s, this was the mainstay of maintaining geometric treatment accuracy. At that time, it was the best technology that was available. However, it presented several problems.

1) The images were 2D, so to determine any 3D corrections required to the patient setup to eliminate any errors, orthogonal images were needed.

2) The radiation dose delivered to tissues could be relatively high—1–3 cGy per image depending on the treatment site.

3) The beam producing the image was in the MV range, meaning that the predominant interaction process was the Compton effect, which is independent of the atomic number of the tissue traversed, whereas when imaging with a diagnostic kV beam, the photoelectric effect is far more prevalent (section 2.4). MV image production relies solely on differences in tissue density, resulting in a much lower contrast image, which could be quite difficult to interpret, especially for the treatment of pelvic tumours.

4) The final shortcoming of MV imaging, referring to point 3) is that it effectively provided guidance on matching bony anatomy, *not* soft tissue. This was particularly a problem for tumours of the thorax and pelvis where organ and hence tumour motion may of concern.

From the mid-2000s, linear accelerators started to be fitted with a diagnostic kV energy X-ray source, together with its own silicon imaging panel, mounted orthogonally to the treatment head and imaging system.

When using a kV beam, it was possible to generate much higher contrast 2D images than the MV system and this option was and still is certainly available. However, a much more widespread use of these systems is to generate a 3D CT dataset of the patient, known as a CBCT imaging. The introduction of CBCT into clinical practice represented a significant quality improvement in terms of the accuracy and precision of radiotherapy delivery and is discussed in more detail in sections 10.2–10.4.

15.5 **Adaptive radiotherapy**

The ability to perform daily CBCT imaging with the possibility of assessing tumour changes (usually, but not always, shrinkage) and anatomical (e.g. weight) changes in the patient raises the possibility of what is termed adaptive radiotherapy, whereby the treatment plan is modified during a treatment course to account for systematic changes in tumour size or patient anatomy that cannot be managed simply by moving the couch, as discussed in section 10.7. An idealized service might offer a range of treatment plans for a specific patient, so that the radiographers could select the best one based on an assessment of pre-treatment CBCT images—what has been termed the 'plan of the day approach'.

In the mid-2010s, a national radiotherapy trial used this approach for bladder cancer. On the basis of two CT planning scans taken 30 minutes apart, participating centres were required to produce three treatment plans from which a plan of the day could be selected by the treatment team on the basis of a pre-treatment CBCT image.

15.6 **Legal framework**

The recommendations of publications such as TSRT are very much professional guidance and there is no explicit legal obligation to adopt them. However, if a serious incident were to occur that could have been prevented by their implementation, it is likely that there would be an uncomfortable discussion to be had with the relevant authorities.

The Ionising Radiation Regulations (IRR) (2017) states that employers must 'make arrangements for a suitable quality assurance programme to be provided in respect of the equipment or apparatus for the purpose of ensuring that it remains capable of restricting so far as is reasonably practicable exposure to the extent that this is compatible with the intended clinical purpose or research objective'.

Again, in respect of equipment, Guidance Notes for The Ionising Radiation (Medical Exposures) Regulations (IR(ME)R) (2017) state:

> Guidelines on acceptable performance criteria for equipment, intended to ensure patient safety, have been produced by scientific professional bodies. The employer may adopt these or similar appropriate criteria. Corrective action should be taken at the earliest opportunity if equipment performance does not meet specified criteria. In some cases where equipment is considered defective, it may be necessary to remove the equipment from service, for example where patient safety could be compromised.

In respect of departmental written procedures and instructions, IRMER requires that employers establish QA programmes for written protocols and procedures—for example, site-specific clinical protocols and work instructions for machine QC checks. Such a QA programme might include who is responsible for writing and authorizing such documents, the formal process for making changes to the document and when the document is next due for review.

Many radiotherapy centres have now introduced software systems to help manage the QMS. There are several commercial systems available, and they are of benefit in, as examples, tracking document revisions, recording acknowledgments that documents have been read and sending out reminders when documents are due for revision. That said, managing a QMS can place significant demands on a service. While a quality manager is usually in place to coordinate activities relating to the QMS, it is the responsibility of all members of the MDT to contribute to it.

15.7 **Audit**

As with quality, the meaning of the term 'audit' within can be quite wide ranging. A quick Google search of 'What is audit?' usually returns hits relating to finance and financial reports of organizations. The Royal College of Radiologists (RCR) defines audit as a tool for improving healthcare and patient outcomes. Audits can be done carried out locally or by an external group. The International Atomic Energy Authority

(IAEA) states that independent external audits are a necessary part of a comprehensive QA programme in radiotherapy.

The following list not exhaustive but indicates what type of audit may be found in radiotherapy centres. It is assumed that the reader will be familiar with clinical audit, which will not be covered specifically here.

15.7.1 Local audit

It is common practice to undertake an audit of processes within radiotherapy on a regular basis. As an example, a member of the physics team may select a few work instructions and talk through the processes they describe with a member of the radiotherapy team (or vice versa). This can be quite an illuminating process for all involved as what may seem obvious to a team which has written the document, may not seem so obvious to a reader from separate, yet closely related discipline. Such reviews may to lead to suggestions for improvements to be incorporated into a subsequent revision.

15.7.2 External audit

External accreditation of an existing quality system is usually renewed every three years. The external accrediting body will visit the site and essentially conduct an audit of the QA system, possibly over several days. They will not only check that written procedures and policies are in date, but that staff are working according to the instructions they contain.

15.7.3 Radiation dose audit

Within the United Kingdom, there exists an Interdepartmental Audit Network. Established and overseen by IPEM, are eight regional audit groups and each radiotherapy centre in the United Kingdom is a member of one group. Each group operates autonomously and arranges an interdepartmental dose audit schedule of group members, usually on an annual basis. Activities undertaken during a dose audit visit may vary from a simple dose check of a linear accelerator to assessment of a VMAT plan in a relatively complex phantom. The key factor is that the measurements are taken with dosimetry equipment that belongs to the visiting centre, that is it is independent from the centre being audited. Often audits may be timed to check a newly installed linear accelerator or treatment planning system before they enter clinical use.

15.7.4 Clinical trials

Clinical trials play a significant role in evaluating the effectiveness of new treatment strategies and in radiotherapy, and they often require new treatment techniques to be used. Most clinical trials in radiotherapy are multi-centre and for the clinical outcomes to be meaningful, quality assurance measures must be in place to make ensure the uniformity of planning and delivery across all participating centres.

In the United Kingdom, the Radiotherapy Trials Quality Assurance (RTTQA) group (<http://www.rttrialsqa.org.uk>) states in its vision statement that it 'provide[s] centrally co-ordinated radiotherapy quality assurance for all relevant trials to eliminate systematic variation in radiotherapy delivery'.

This is primarily achieved by the provision of:

1) a baseline questionnaire to determine staffing and equipment levels with the participating centre;

2) a trial-specific questionnaire which often requests a process document within which each centre should identify how it will fulfil the trial requirements for treatment planning, delivery, and verification;

3) image datasets on which clinicians are required to define target volumes and organs at risk. There is always at least one planning CT dataset, which is often supplemented with MR images and a brief medical history to inform the contouring process;

4) image datasets—usually with predefined volumes—on which a treatment plan can be produced to meet the trial dose criteria;

5) a site visit to participating centres to audit the planning and delivery processes and measure doses in a phantom to compare those calculated in the treatment planning system.

15.8 **Incident reporting and risk**

The following statement may sound alarming, but incidents in radiotherapy are not uncommon. However, the significant majority are relatively minor. TSRT defines five levels of incident, these being:

♦ Level 1—a serious radiation incident, reportable to the CQC under IRMER 2017;

♦ Level 2—non-reportable radiation incident. A non-reportable radiation incident is defined as a radiation incident which is not reportable, but of potential or actual clinical significance;

♦ Level 3—minor radiation incident. A minor radiation incident is defined as a radiation incident in the technical sense, but of no potential or actual clinical significance;

♦ Level 4—near miss. A near miss is defined as a potential radiation incident that was detected and prevented before treatment delivery;

♦ Level 5—other non-conformance classed as a non-conformity, detected as part of a checking process.

The largest numbers of incidents are usually levels 4 and 5. It is important that all incidents are reviewed by an MDT regularly to pick up patterns or trends. Repeated incidents with the same cause may, for example, highlight a training need or improved clarity in work instructions. The outcomes of incidents should be fed back to the MDT to help facilitate quality improvements. Such incident data are also submitted to a central agency for national reporting.

15.9 **Significant radiotherapy incidents**

Or: What happens when quality fails?

Since the late 1980s, there have been several serious radiotherapy incidents in the United Kingdom which have led to changes in practice and quality improvements. In chronological order, they have been as follows.

15.9.1 **1988 Cobalt miscalibration**

A cobalt source was changed in a teletherapy unit at the start of 1988. A physicist measured the output of unit in terms of Grays/minute to determine appropriate treatment times before it re-entered clinical use. The dosimetry equipment used went 'off-scale' when used for 1 minute so the physicist measured for 0.8 minute instead. Unfortunately, the dose readings obtained were not scaled for this shorter measuring period, so all subsequent treatments delivered a 25% overdose to patients. (1 min/0.8 min = +25%).

The error was found later in the year during an external dose audit. An independent inquiry stated that 207 patients had received an overdose and in 10 cases, this overdose was considered life threatening. A subsequent report by the DoH 'Quality Assurance in Radiotherapy' authored by Bleehan in 1994 recommended departments implement a quality assurance programme based on the international standard, ISO900. This incident also highlighted the importance of external dose audit.

15.9.2 **1991 Monitor unit calculation process error**

A new TPS was commissioned in a department. During the commissioning procedure, it was discovered that while the preceding TPS had been calculating treatment monitor units correctly, the planning team had been applying legacy inverse square corrections for isocentric-type treatments, in addition to the corrections applied by the TPS. This had resulted in an under dose to patients treated isocentrically by a magnitude dependent on the focus-to-surface (FSD) difference from 100 cm.

For example, for an isocentric beam with an FSD of 90 cm, the under dose would have been approximately $90^2/100^2$ or around 20%. With an FSD of 85 cm, the underdose would have been just under 30%.

An independent review found that over a period of nearly a decade, 1045 patients had received an under dose to some degree and approximately 600 patients were under dosed by 21–30%.

It was noted, somewhat fortunately, that isocentric type treatments were not in common use at the centre during this period. It was concluded that poorly designed management lines resulted in no-one being authorized as responsible for undertaking such quality control checks that might have succeeded in detecting this error at an earlier stage.

15.9.3 **2004 Data entry error**

A patient received a dose of approximately 100 Gy following the omission of a planned wedge from a beam during the manual preparation of a treatment prescription on a treatment unit. The prescribed MUs were high to account for wedge attenuation, when in fact there was no wedge in the beam. The subsequent independent enquiry recommended that electronic transfer of data should be implemented as soon as possible. The report also highlighted the need to review checking procedures to avoid 'involuntary automaticity'—in this case, essentially seeing what was expected to be seen, rather than what was actually there.

15.9.4 **2006 Treatment planning process error**

A patient was treated for a brain tumour and received a 58% overdose. The underlying cause was found to be that the centre had traditionally planned treatments for a nominal number of MU per Gray and when the treatment was prescribed, a correction was made to the MU to deliver the correct dose for the prescription. However, planning procedures changed and the plan produced in this case had the correct MU for the prescribed treatment. The subsequent enquiry found that the relevant documentation had not been updated in respect of the change of MU calculation and that an independent MU check had not been performed.

A summary of international serious radiotherapy incidents can be found on the IAEA website at:

<https://www.iaea.org/resources/rpop/health-professionals/radiotherapy/accident-prevention>.

15.10 **Summary of the lessons learned from past mistakes**

Electronic transfer, quality systems, commissioning processes, external dosimetry audit, MU checking; all performed from necessity to ensure we do not repeat the past.

Major radiotherapy incidents in the United Kingdom over the past 50 years have been mercifully rare.

The incidents cited above in 1988 and 1991 acted together as a catalyst to kick start the implementation of quality improvements in radiotherapy, beginning with the introduction of quality systems in radiotherapy departments. The 1988 incident also highlighted the importance of external dosimetry audit which has now become standard practice across the United Kingdom.

Subsequent developments such as electronic transfer of plan data, the implementation of image-guided radiotherapy (IGRT) and improved plan checking processes have all contributed to the reduction of risk in the radiotherapy process. However, it would be unwise to assume that all possible sources of error, significant or minor, have now or ever will be eliminated in radiotherapy.

Given the complex nature of treatment planning and delivery with multi-professional interfaces, the possibility of an error occurring always exists and it is important that when it does, a culture of openness and honesty allows such experiences to be widely shared so that sources of the error can be understood, and steps can be taken to stop it recurring.

Closing with a quotation again attributed to Henry Ford: 'The only real mistake is one from which we learn nothing.'

Further reading

Professional guidance

Dose and Volume Specification for Reporting Intracavitary Therapy in Gynecology, ICRU Report 38, Bethesda, MD: ICRU, 1985.

Prescribing, Recording, and Reporting Photon Beam Therapy, ICRU Report 50, Bethesda, MD: ICRU, 1993.

Prescribing, Recording and Reporting Photon Beam Therapy, ICRU Report 62, Bethesda, MD: ICRU, 1999.

Prescribing, Recording, and Reporting Electron Beam Therapy, ICRU Report 71, Bethesda, MD: ICRU, 2004.

Prescribing, Recording, and Reporting Intensity-Modulated Photon-Beam Therapy (IMRT), ICRU Report 83, Bethesda, MD: ICRU, 2010.

The Royal College of Radiologists, Towards Safer Radiotherapy. BFCO(08)1. London, UK: The Royal College of Radiologists, 2008. Available from: <https://www.rcr.ac.uk/system/files/publication/field_publication_files/Towards_saferRT_final.pdf>

The Royal College of Radiologists, Guidance on IRMER Implications for Clinical Practice in Radiotherapy. London, UK: The Royal College of Radiologists 2020. Available from: <https://www.rcr.ac.uk/sites/default/files/guidance-on-irmer-implications-for-clinical-practice-in-radiotherapy.pdf>

The Department of Health and Social Care, June 2018, Guidance to the Ionising Radiation (Medical Exposure) Regulations 2017. The Department of Health and Social Care. Available from: <https://assets.publishing.service.gov.uk/government/uploads/system/uploads/attachment_data/file/720282/guidance-to-the-ionising-radiation-medical-exposure-regulations-2017.pdf>

European Society for Radiotherapy and Oncology (ESTRO), Brachytherapy Guidelines. A number of useful guidelines on brachytherapy are available from: <https://www.estro.org/Science/Guidelines>

Statutory regulations

The Ionising Radiation Regulations (IRR) 2017 (Statutory Instrument 2017, No 1075) London, UK: HMSO 2017. Available from <https://www.legislation.gov.uk/uksi/2017/1075/contents/made>

The Ionising Radiation (Medical Exposure) Regulations 2017 (IRMER) (Statutory Instrument 2017 No 1322) London, UK: HMSO 2017. Available from <https://www.legislation.gov.uk/uksi/2017/1322/made>

Physics texts

Faiz M. Khan (ed). The Physics of Radiation Therapy, 6th edn. Philadelphia, PA: Lippincott, Williams and Wilkins, 2019.

Philip Mayles, Alan E. Nahum, and J.C. Rosenwald (eds). *Handbook of Radiotherapy Physics Theory and Practice*, 2nd edn. London: Taylor and Francis, 2020.

Other *Radiotherapy in Practice* titles

Peter Hoskin (ed). *Radiotherapy in Practice—Radioisotope Therapy*, 2nd edn. Oxford: Oxford University Press, 2007.

Peter Hoskin (ed). *Radiotherapy In Practice—External Beam Therapy*, 3rd edn. Oxford: Oxford University Press, 2019.

Peter Hoskin and Catherine Coyle (eds). *Radiotherapy In Practice—Brachytherapy*, 2nd edn. Oxford: Oxford University Press, 2011.

Peter Hoskin, Thankammer Ajithkumar, and Vicky Goh (eds). *Radiotherapy In Practice—Imaging for Clinical Oncology*, 2nd edn. Oxford: Oxford University Press, 2021.

Index

For the benefit of digital users, indexed terms that span two pages (e.g., 52–53) may, on occasion, appear on only one of those pages.

Tables and boxes are indicated by *t* and *b* following the page number